SO-EDI-720

New Drug
Treatments
for
Diabetes

Dana Armstrong, R.D., C.D.E., and
Allen Bennett King, M.D., F.A.C.P., F.A.C.E.

Publications International, Ltd.

Dana Armstrong, R.D., C.D.E., received her degree in nutrition and dietetics from the University of California, Davis. She has been in private practice for 15 years and has developed an educational program that has benefited more than 2,000 patients with diabetes. She is the cofounder and program director of the Diabetes Care Center in Salinas, California. She specializes in and speaks nationally on the use of nondiet approaches to disease treatment, specifically diabetes. Having a child with diabetes, she combines her professional knowledge with personal experience and understanding.

Allen Bennett King, M.D., F.A.C.P., F.A.C.E., received his degrees and training at the University of California, Berkeley; Creighton University Medical School; the University of Colorado; and Stanford University. He has authored more than 20 papers in medical science and speaks nationally on new advances in diabetes. Over his 32 years of practice he has seen more than 5,000 patients with diabetes, some for more than 25 years. He is an assistant clinical professor at the University of California Natividad Medical Center, cofounder and medical director of the Diabetes Care Center in Salinas, California, and the son of Earle King, who died in 1978 from the complications of diabetes.

Together, in October 1998, Dana Armstrong and Allen King opened a private practice focused on the treatment, education, and support of people with diabetes. Their philosophy is to empower patients who have diabetes with knowledge and education that lets patients control their health, life, and future.

Contents

Choose Wisely

In 1968, my father, Earle King, came home from his doctor's visit with a prescription for Tolinase, a commonly used diabetic medication at that time, and a one-page diet instruction sheet for reducing calories and eliminating sugar from his diet. He gave it to my mother, who posted it on the inside of the cupboard door, never to be read again.

Needless to say, the diet was not followed, Tolinase never did control his blood sugar, and his blood fats and blood pressure problems were never addressed. Ten years later, my father died from the complications of diabetic kidney disease compounded by carotid and coronary artery disease. (The carotid arteries in the neck supply blood to the head, and the coronary arteries supply blood to the heart.) I often wonder, with the improvements in diabetes treatment and care, would this happen today? We don't think so. We think that *no one* should have complications—let alone die—from diabetes today.

The purpose of this book is to educate and empower you so that you can determine what you want and what to expect from your health care provider and yourself. It is within your power to prevent the devastating problems that can result from uncontrolled diabetes. And the many recent advances in drug treatments, monitoring, and other therapies that you'll learn about in this book can help greatly.

Each chapter will give you a greater understanding of your diabetes, and through this understanding you will gain the power and confidence to care for yourself. The first chapters will give you the background of "how" diabetes works and exactly what is going on inside of your body. The next chapters detail some of the proactive measures you can take to better manage your diabetes, such as testing your blood glucose levels regularly; having an active, playful life; and eating with joy, pleasure, and gusto. The final chapters of the book are dedicated to leading you through the maze of medications that have recently become available to help you and your diabetes care team treat your diabetes effectively. By putting all of this information to use, you will feel confident in taking that important step toward caring for your own diabetes instead of relying solely on your health care professional. By gaining knowledge, you will become a strong advocate of better diabetes care for yourself, your family, and your community. The outlook for successfully controlling diabetes and living free of diabetes complications has never been better. But you must make the choice and the effort to reach for that healthier future. Join us in taking the first step.

CHAPTER 1

What Is Diabetes, Anyway?

To get the most from the latest advances and proven treatments in diabetes care, you need to understand what it means to have diabetes. A good place to start is learning how the body uses fuel and how that process goes awry in diabetes.

Getting to Know Glucose

Even if you've only recently been diagnosed with diabetes, you've probably already heard the term *glucose*. It is an important player in the body and in diabetes.

In your bloodstream, circulating to all the organs of your body, is sugar. Most of the sugar in your body is the kind called glucose. (Other sugars in your body include fructose, the sugar found in fruit, and ribose, a sugar that makes up the chromosomes that carry your genetic information.) Glucose's main job is to supply the body with energy. The body breaks down glucose, releasing energy, water, and carbon dioxide, the gas we expel when we exhale.

Glucose is a quickly available fuel source that can be used by nearly all of the tissues in the body. And when it comes to your brain, glucose is the *only* source of fuel it can use. The brain can survive without glucose for only a short time, just as it can go for only a few minutes without oxygen. Because glucose is the only fuel your brain can use, your brain directs your nervous system and hormone-producing glands to protect your glucose level, making sure it does not fall too low. It is the glucose level that is meant when people talk about blood sugar, and it is the glucose level in your blood that is affected by diabetes.

The other fuel used in the body are the *fatty acids*. Fatty acids differ from glucose in that they provide a source of fuel that is called upon only during longer periods of fasting. Fatty acids come from the fat we eat, and they are stored in our fat cells as *triglycerides*. Triglycerides are continuously being converted into fatty acids in the blood and then back again, waiting to be called upon for energy. The more fatty acids we store away in our fat cells, the more "visible" our energy reserves become. Excesses of these fatty acids are now found to play a role in the development of diabetes and are discussed in more detail in Chapter 4.

Getting Glucose
Where It Needs to Go

The glucose in your body comes from three major nutrients: fats, proteins, and carbohydrates. About 10 percent of the fat and 50 percent of the protein you eat is eventually broken down into glucose (the rest is used for other purposes or stored in the body's fat cells), but nearly 100 percent of the carbohydrates you eat are broken down into glucose. Chewing your food and drinking liquids begins the digestive process of breaking starches and larger sugar molecules down to glucose. The enzymes found in your mouth and throughout your intestines complete the breakdown. The glucose is then absorbed into the bloodstream and travels throughout the body.

This process requires help from your *pancreas*. The pancreas is an organ about the size of your fist that lies just behind your stomach. One of the jobs of the pancreas is to make enzymes for food digestion. But the pancreas also plays another important role. The pancreas contains small groups of cells, called the *islets of Langerhans*, which make hormones that are released into your bloodstream. Some 80 percent of these islet cells are *beta cells*. Beta cells make a small protein molecule—the hormone *insulin*.

Insulin plays many important roles in the body, but its primary task is to cause the tissues to take in proteins, fatty acids, and glucose. Insulin is like a key that opens a door on the body's cells, so the nutrients needed by the cells can get inside. When a person who does not have diabetes eats any food, their blood glucose level rises; the beta cells in the pancreas detect this rise and release more insulin. The insulin goes to the liver, telling it to make less glucose, and to the muscles and fat cells, telling them to take up more glucose. This allows the nutrients from the recently eaten food to enter and "feed" the body's cells, it keeps the blood glucose level from rising too high even after eating, and it allows the blood glucose level to quickly return to a normal, healthy range. When that same healthy person fasts, such as between meals or during sleep, the insulin levels fall, causing the liver to make more glucose to provide the brain and other organs with energy until the next meal.

In the person with diabetes, this feedback process doesn't work properly. Insulin does not do its job, and the person's blood glucose rises to unhealthy levels.

Detecting Diabetes

In a person who does not have diabetes, the body keeps the *plasma glucose level* (see box below) between meals in the range of 70 to 109 milligrams per deciliter, or mg/dl. After eating, that person's glucose level rises, depending on the amount and content of the meal, but does not exceed 139 mg/dl. It also quickly returns to the fasting, or between-meal, range.

In a person with diabetes, the blood glucose level rises abnormally high after eating, takes much longer to come down, and doesn't settle back into the normal range, even during periods of fasting such as between meals. So in order to diagnose diabetes, a doctor must test your blood glucose levels.

What's *Plasma*?

Throughout this book, *blood glucose level* refers to plasma glucose level unless otherwise noted. The term plasma simply refers to the liquid part of the blood that remains after the blood cells have been removed. It's the portion of blood tested during glucose tests in the laboratory or doctor's office. And the difference between blood glucose and plasma glucose is really only important when choosing and reading personal glucose meters, which are discussed in Chapter 5.

There are actually three different tests that can be used to determine if you have diabetes. The most common method used to diagnose diabetes is a blood test in which your *fasting plasma glucose* is measured. A fasting test means it has been more than eight hours since you have had anything to eat. When your fasting plasma glucose is over 125 mg/dl on two consecutive occasions, a diagnosis of diabetes is made.

Another method used to diagnosis diabetes is a *random blood glucose test*. This is a glucose test taken without regard to how long it has been since you have eaten. If your

Remember!

Warning symptoms of diabetes include frequent urination, excessive thirst, excessive hunger, unexplained weight loss, and fatigue.

random blood glucose value is 200 mg/dl or higher and you have symptoms of diabetes—such as frequent urination, excessive thirst, excessive hunger, weight loss, or fatigue—the diagnosis of diabetes is made.

The third test is an *oral glucose tolerance test*. This test is done when a test of the fasting blood glucose shows a level close to normal but diabetes is suspected (because, for example, the above-mentioned symptoms of diabetes are present). An oral glucose tolerance test is given after three days of a diet high in starches and sugars. After an overnight fast, you arrive at the lab for a two-hour test. Your blood is drawn to measure your fasting plasma level. You are then asked to drink a high-glucose-concentration liquid over a 15-minute period. During the remainder of the time, your blood is drawn at specified intervals. It is important to sit for the entire test and report if you feel ill during the test. Diabetes is diagnosed if your blood glucose level exceeds 199 mg/dl during the test.

You may have noticed that there's a gap between a glucose level that's considered normal and one that indicates diabetes. A normal fasting glucose level, for example, is less than 110 mg/dl, but it's

Making the Diagnosis

TYPE OF TEST:	FASTING BLOOD GLUCOSE (FBG)	RANDOM BLOOD GLUCOSE (RBG)	ORAL GLUCOSE TOLERANCE
It is **diabetes** when:	FBG ≥125 mg/dl on two consecutive blood tests	RBG ≥200 mg/dl, plus diabetes symptoms	2-hour glucose level ≥200 mg/dl
It is **impaired glucose tolerance** when:	FBG ≥110 mg/dl and <125 mg/dl		2-hour glucose level is ≥140 mg/dl and <200 mg/dl
It is **normal** when:	FBG <110 mg/dl		

only when the fasting glucose level rises above 125 mg/dl that a diagnosis of diabetes is made. Likewise, at the end of a two-hour glucose tolerance test, a normal glucose level should be less than 140 mg/dl, and yet a diagnosis of diabetes isn't made unless the glucose level after those two hours is 200 mg/dl or higher. What about the range in between?

Glucose levels of 110 to 124 mg/dl when fasting and two-hour glucose levels of 140 to 199 mg/dl are not considered diabetes but are not normal, either. People with these levels are diagnosed as having *impaired glucose tolerance*. Although not yet considered to have diabetes, these people have a 25 percent chance of developing diabetes in the future and also have a higher incidence of heart disease.

Different Kinds of Diabetes

Once the diagnosis of diabetes is made, the next task is to determine what type of diabetes you have. There are four types of diabetes: Type 1 diabetes, Type 2 diabetes, gestational diabetes, and secondary diabetes. Each type of diabetes requires a different treatment approach.

TYPE 1 DIABETES Type 1 diabetes affects about five percent of all people who have diabetes. It is sometimes referred to as *juvenile diabetes* because there is a higher rate of diagnosis in children between the ages of 10 and 14, but people of any age group can develop Type 1 diabetes. It may also be called *insulin-dependent diabetes*, because diabetes pills are ineffective in treating the high blood glucose level; these individuals require injections of insulin to control their blood glucose. (As you will learn shortly, a small number of people with Type 1 who are in the very earliest stages of the disease may not yet require insulin; eventually, however, they will.)

Type 1 diabetes is a disease of "dumb" white blood cells. Normally, white blood cells are responsible for recognizing foreign objects in our blood and then attacking these foreign objects with antibodies. In Type 1 diabetes, the white cells believe the beta cells of the pancreas do not belong there. An inflammation ensues, and the antibodies attack the beta cells. This destruction of beta cells can happen either very quickly or slowly over a long period of time. When enough beta cells are lost, insulin deficiency develops and blood glucose levels begin to rise. Occasionally you can identify the viral infection that set off the attack, but generally no such illness can be identified. To make things more complicated, it is not always possible to identify the presence of anti-bodies (the marker of autoimmunity) in the blood. This is especially common in African and Chinese Americans. In these racial groups, and in some other groups of people, there is probably another cause for the malfunctioning of the beta cells, but this reason has not yet been discovered.

In Type 1 diabetes, there is a chance of developing *ketoacidosis* because of the extreme lack of insulin. The lack of enough insulin makes it hard for your body to use glucose for energy. If your body cannot get glucose from your blood, it breaks down fat to supply energy to your cells. When this happens, ketones, which are more acidic than normal body tissues, accumulate in the blood. Ketones are normally removed from the blood by your kidneys and passed out of your body in urine. When more ketones are produced than your kidneys can handle, excess ketones build up in the blood. If not treated, this can lead to ketoacidosis, an extremely serious and life-threatening condition. This situation may lead to diabetic coma and death.

Your disease is most likely Type 1 if you develop diabetes before age 35, are lean, have a family history of diabetes treated with insulin, and require insulin injections. Additional tests may be done to confirm the diagnosis. These tests include measuring islet-cell antibodies (the antibodies directed toward destroying the islet cells), C-peptide level (a measurement of the amount of insulin being made by the body), and urine ketones. A positive islet-cell antibody test, a low C-peptide level, or the presence of ketones in the urine all suggest a diagnosis of Type 1 diabetes.

If you have Type 1 diabetes, you probably will require insulin to control your glucose. However, the occasional person in the earliest stages

Type Casting

Although diabetes that develops before age 35 is likely to be the Type 1 variety, more and more overweight children are developing Type 2 diabetes.

of Type 1 may still have some islet cells left that secrete enough insulin so that insulin injections are not yet required. Pills or changes in diet, activity, and lifestyle may be enough to control blood glucose. Still, because the person has Type 1 diabetes, their white blood cells are still attacking their islet cells, and the insulin-making beta cells are slowly being destroyed. So, with time, insulin injections will become necessary. Ongoing clinical trials are currently looking at using injections of small doses of insulin early in this diagnosis phase as a sort of decoy. It is hoped the white blood cells will be distracted by the foreign insulin, taking them off the attack of the islet cells and thus preserving insulin production in the body for a longer period of time.

TYPE 2 DIABETES Type 2 diabetes is the most common form of diabetes, and it is the subject of this book. It is estimated that up to 90 percent of the people with diabetes have the Type 2 form. The cause of Type 2 diabetes appears to be resistance to insulin's action and/or a deficiency of insulin secretion. But how does one separate it from Type 1 diabetes? Type 2 diabetes almost never causes ketoacidosis and shows no evidence of autoimmunity (in other words, there are no signs of antibodies attacking the islet cells). People with Type 2 diabetes usually are over age 35, are overweight, and have a family history of diabetes treated with diet or pills. Still, distinguishing between Type 1 and Type 2 diabetes can be very difficult. Indeed, it has been found that almost five percent of adults who are diagnosed as having Type 2 diabetes actually have Type 1. Furthermore, the incidence of Type 2 diabetes in childhood is rapidly increasing in frequency. That makes the automatic diagnosis of Type 1 diabetes in children more confusing as well.

The disease of Type 2 diabetes begins decades before diagnosis, with an increasing resistance to insulin. This increasing resistance is the result of genetics, weight gain (especially abdominal fat), decreased activity, and aging. The major site of insulin resistance is the muscles. The muscles normally use more than 80 percent of the glucose that is taken into the body, so it is the muscles that are the major site of insulin resistance. Because of this resistance to insulin, the insulin levels in the body actually begin to increase. In an attempt to make up for the diminished effective-ness of the insulin, the body cranks up insulin production. For reasons not entirely clear, in those people destined for diabetes, the beta cells slowly begin to fail to keep up with the demand for insulin. They get burned out, in a sense. At first, the plasma glucose level begins to rise above

What Type of Diabetes Do I Have?

CHARACTERISTICS	TYPE 1 DIABETES	TYPE 2 DIABETES
Age of onset	younger than 35	older than 35
Need insulin	yes	no
Family history of diabetes	infrequent	usually
Big belly	no	yes
Ketones in urine	yes	no

normal after meals, and then eventually the fasting glucose levels begin to remain above normal as well. When the glucose levels rise high enough to produce symptoms, or when an accompanying complication, such as a heart attack, sends the patient to the hospital, the diagnosis of Type 2 diabetes is made.

GESTATIONAL DIABETES Gestational diabetes means that the diabetes is diagnosed for the first time during pregnancy. Gestational diabetes occurs in about three percent of all pregnancies. Gestational diabetes is diagnosed using a three-hour glucose tolerance test. If the glucose levels exceed any two of the upper limits of normal, the diagnosis is made. Rarely are the glucose levels elevated enough to harm the mother. The problem is that the mother's blood glucose flows freely into the growing fetus's blood. The fetus, in turn, releases insulin from its own pancreas to lower its own glucose levels. This forces glucose into the fetus's tissues, causing it to become large for its gestational age and resulting in a difficult labor and delivery. The increase in glucose appears to be due to a lack of insulin release or a resistance to insulin's action that was present in the mother before becoming pregnant. During pregnancy, the placenta releases high amounts of hormones that further decrease the effectiveness of the mother's insulin. This causes her blood glucose levels to increase. Since the placenta grows as the pregnancy progresses and continues to put out more and more hormones, the mother's insulin resistance increases and glucose levels rise higher and higher, right up to the time of delivery. With the delivery of the baby and the removal of the placenta, however, the glucose levels promptly return to normal in up to 97 percent of these women.

By making modifications in their diets and increasing their activity levels, many

Studying Up

Researchers are currently studying the feasibility of using pills—rather than insulin—to treat gestational diabetes.

women are able to control the rising glucose levels during their pregnancies. For some, however, the insulin resistance is too great. These women require the use of insulin, generally prior to all meals and before going to bed, to keep glucose levels within a healthy range for the baby. New studies now underway are looking at the use of pills instead of insulin to control the glucose levels in women with gestational diabetes, but the results are not yet in.

Gestational diabetes is often viewed as a window into the future. Women who have had gestational diabetes have a significantly higher chance of developing diabetes sometime in the future, at a general rate of about three percent each year. A few studies have shown that weight control and increased physical activity may lessen the chance for future diabetes by 50 percent. There are even studies currently underway to evaluate the ability of some of the new diabetes pills to prevent future diabetes in women who have had gestational diabetes.

SECONDARY DIABETES Secondary diabetes is seen in about three percent of all people with diabetes. Secondary means the diabetes is secondary to another cause. Potential causes include medications that harm the pancreas or interfere with insulin's action, damage to the pancreas from alcohol abuse, or a cancer or hormone problem that affects blood glucose. Although many patients with diabetes have conditions or take medications that may aggravate their glucose levels, seldom are these factors the major cause of diabetes.

Can My Children Get My Diabetes?

About 20 percent of Americans between the ages of 40 and 75 years of age have diabetes, and about half of them do not even know they have the disease. Certain ethnic groups have an even higher incidence of diabetes; these include African, Asian, and Hispanic Americans; Pacific Islanders; and Native Americans. Indeed, in some American Indian tribes, eight out of every ten tribe members have diabetes. Further, the prevalence of diabetes in the United States is increasing due to the aging of the population in general, the change in ethnic mix toward a greater percentage of susceptible people, increasing obesity, and decreasing physical activity.

Type 2 diabetes is inherited as a dominant trait. This means that if you have diabetes, your children have at least a one-in-four chance of developing the disease. Those people who have been diagnosed usually have some relative who also has the disease. But contrary to popular myth, diabetes does not skip generations. The chart on page 23 can also help you to evaluate your risk of developing Type 2 diabetes.

Why Should I Bother to Control My Glucose?

When your blood glucose level increases to 180 mg/dl or more, the excess glucose spills over into your urine, causing you to urinate more frequently and, consequently, increasing your thirst. Because your body's cells cannot take in and use the glucose in your blood, they become starved for fuel. This makes you feel hungry and fatigued, and you become unusually sleepy, especially after a meal. If your blood glucose levels remain above 180, the white blood cells in your body do not work as well as they should, leaving you more vulnerable to infections. Any wounds you receive become slow to heal, and you are more likely to get bladder and yeast infections. The yeast infections commonly will not get better until your blood glucose levels return to normal. If your blood glucose levels continue to remain above 180, the glucose becomes increasingly toxic to your body. As a result, severe damage begins to occur in your eyes, kidneys, feet, and heart.

That's only a brief description of the kinds of changes that untreated diabetes can cause in your body (you'll find more details in Chapter 3). But you can take steps to forestall the frightening consequences of high blood glucose. Treating your diabetes means getting control not only of your blood glucose but your life. You need to become educated about diabetes, pay more attention to what is happening in your life and in your body, and start living in awareness. You can take charge. Indeed, you are the only one who can make the choice to take care of yourself. Read on to find out how trained professionals and the best of standard and new medical treatments can help.

CHAPTER 2

Take Command of Your Care

he latest approach to diabetes treatment puts you in charge of your own care. You become the boss of your diabetes team, hiring the staff that best serves your needs, tracking your prog- ress, and keeping your eyes on the ulti- mate goal—your health and well-being.

Assemble Your Staff

Getting the best treatment for your diabetes is not simply a matter of keeping your doctor's appoint- ments and taking pills. Diabetes affects many aspects of your life. And since nobody knows your life better than you do, you must step into the role of the "general" of your diabetes care in order to get your treatment needs met.

As the general, you'll want to surround yourself with knowledgeable, trustworthy, expert "advi- sors"—your diabetes care team—who can help you get the information, advice, treatments, and support you need to manage your diabetes effectively. This team is usually composed of your doctor, diabetes educator, dietitian, pharmacist, and dentist. It may also include a mental-health professional, a podiatrist (foot doctor), and a cardiologist (heart specialist). As you go about assembling your team, remember that these people work for *you*. You are hiring them to help you learn about diabetes, understand how it specifically affects you, and provide you with the tools that let you make your own informed health care decisions.

Your first task is to find a doctor. You'll not only want a physician who has skill and experience in diagnosing and treating diabetes, but also one who will support and work with you in becoming your own diabetes general. Together you and your doctor need to develop a good working relationship where there is mutual understanding, respect, and trust. You will need to feel comfortable talking with and asking questions of your doctor. If you are unable to develop such a relationship, you need to find another doctor.

There are many diabetes specialists, and you can get a list of the doctors in your area by contacting your local chapter of the American Diabetes Association (see Resources). You can also call your local medical society and ask for a list of doctors who are "board certified" in endocrinology (the specialty that focuses on hormonal disorders, such as diabetes), internal medicine, or family practice. If you cannot find a specialist near you, pick a primary care doctor who will work with you and who will not hesitate to refer you to a specialist when one might be needed.

Education is by far the most basic tool of diabetes care. It involves learning how to take care of yourself and your diabetes, and it brings you into the decision-making process for your own health. So after you find a doctor, you'll need to add a diabetes educator to your team.

> ### Get Smart
> Education is the most basic tool in diabetes care, so add a diabetes educator to your team.

The diabetes educator will provide you with information and one-on-one guidance. As with your doctor, the educator you choose should be someone you feel comfortable talking to and someone you feel you can contact with questions about the practical details of diabetes care.

Most often, a diabetes educator will also be a nurse, dietitian, or pharmacist by training. If possible, choose a certified diabetes educator, or CDE. A CDE is a health professional who is certified by the National Certification Board for Diabetes Educators to teach people with diabetes how to manage the disease. CDEs must have at least two years' experience in diabetes education, must have successfully completed a comprehensive examination covering diabetes, and must retake the national examination every five years to remain certified. Your physician may be able to recommend a diabetes educator, or you can contact the American Association of Diabetes Educators (see Resources) for the names of diabetes educators near you.

With the help of your doctor and diabetes educator, you should be able to get additional referrals to a dentist, eye doctor, podiatrist, and cardiologist if needed. If you already have an established relationship with a dentist or eye doctor, be sure to discuss your diabetes diagnosis with them and perhaps even put them in touch with the other members of your team so that they can collaborate on your care.

Focus on Taking Control

Being diagnosed with diabetes and then being told to alter your life can spark some pretty intense emotions. It's natural to feel stressed, afraid, sad, or even angry at the news that you have the disease. But while such reactions may be normal, they can be harmful if you don't work through them and then refocus your energy into taking care of yourself and your diabetes.

For some people, the stress of a diabetes diagnosis can turn into denial. Testing your blood glucose level simply becomes a constant reminder that you have diabetes. So by not checking your blood glucose levels, you begin to feel as if you really don't have the disease. To further the denial, you attribute your symptoms of high glucose levels, such as excessive thirst and fatigue, to some other cause, such as the hot weather or working long hours. Perhaps you cancel or just don't show up for your medical appointments. Ignoring the fact that you have diabetes will not make it go away. People who live in denial about their diabetes die.

Fear, too, is a common reaction to the stress of dealing with diabetes. Perhaps you know or have heard of someone who is suffering from multiple, crippling complications from diabetes or may have even died of diabetes complications. While it makes sense to fear the complications of diabetes, do not let that fear paralyze you. Indeed, use the fear of diabetes complications as strong motivation for learning all that you can about your disease and working hard to gain the best possible control of your blood glucose levels.

Feeling sad or down is yet another common reaction to a diabetes diagnosis as well as an occasional response to the stress of coping with the disease. When that blue feeling lasts more than a few weeks or really begins to interfere with your daily life or with taking care of your diabetes, it may be depression. While depression is more common among people with diabetes, it can be treated. Depression is a biochemical condition. It is not a defect in your character. Depression is associated with an imbalance of brain hormones,

Are You Depressed?

Ask yourself the following questions, and check off those items you've experienced nearly every day, all day, for at least two weeks.

I feel sad or down in the dumps. _____

I feel worthless and guilty. _____

I have trouble concentrating, remembering, or making decisions. _____

I'm experiencing changes in my appetite or unexpected changes in my weight. _____

I feel tired and lack energy all the time. _____

I don't care much about things I used to enjoy. _____

I'm not particularly interested in sex. _____

I have trouble sleeping or I've been sleeping more than usual. _____

I have frequent headaches. _____

I have frequent aches and pains. _____

I have digestive troubles. _____

I feel pessimistic and hopeless. _____

I'm anxious and worried. _____

I feel slow and lethargic or I feel restless and can't seem to sit still. _____

I find myself crying for no good reason. _____

If you have checked several items, you may be depressed and should talk to your doctor. If you are having or have had any thoughts about suicide, contact a health professional or hospital immediately.

and once these hormones are corrected with therapy and/or medications, your mood and functioning will improve.

The quiz on the previous page can help you assess whether you may be depressed. If you suspect that you are suffering from depression, discuss it with your doctor. Your doctor may choose from many available medications and/or may refer you to a psychotherapist, psychologist, or psychiatrist.

Chart Your Own Course

Charting your own course is not just a figure of speech. As the general in charge of your diabetes care, you should create your own chart, much like the kind a doctor keeps. This way, you can have all the information about your disease in one place, and you can take it with you each time you meet with a member of your diabetes-care team.

In this chart, you should keep a complete listing of your medical conditions and all of your medications, copies of all of your lab-test results (get a copy at each visit or ask the laboratory to send you a copy), any informational handouts or instructions from your team, a list of the names and contact information for all the members of your diabetes care team, and a list of any questions you may have about your diabetes. You can even include calendar sheets with all your medical appointments noted.

It is of crucial importance that your chart include a complete and accurate list of all your medications and the strength and dose of each one. Be sure to include all of your prescription items as well as any nonprescription medicines, vitamins, minerals, and herbs you take. You may be seeing more than one doctor, and it is important that each one knows what the other has prescribed for you and what over-the-counter products you take so that together you can avoid dangerous interactions. It is also important for *you* to know what you are taking, why you are taking it, and what side effects or warning signs may occur. It is, after all, your body, and you shouldn't put anything in it that you don't understand. Be sure to note in your chart any side effects or unusual symptoms that you suspect may be connected to your medications. This way you can inquire about them the next time you talk to your doctor.

It's also very helpful to make a running list of questions you have about diabetes so that you can ask your team. Jot them down as they occur to you. Often, under the pressure of limited time or nervousness during the appointment, you can easily forget questions that otherwise seemed so

What Your Own Medical Chart Should Include

A list of your medicines, strengths and doses, and who prescribed them

A list of your medical conditions and dates of diagnosis, any allergies to medications, and all major medical events and surgeries

A listing of all your doctors and health care professionals and their emergency phone numbers

A section for placing your laboratory results and any handouts, information sheets, and instructions given to you by your diabetes care team

A list of questions you have for your doctor or health care professional

A copy of this book!

clear in your mind the previous day. Also, prioritize your questions so the most important question is answered first. If you are unable to complete your list, inform your doctor so that you can make another appointment to get answers to the remainder of your questions.

Make sure to prepare for each visit the night before the appointment. Don't forget to bring your chart as well as your blood glucose meter and your log books (you'll learn more about meters and log books in upcoming chapters).

Remember, you are the general in charge of your care. Take time to focus and assemble the personnel and resources you need to accomplish your mission. That mission—taking care of your diabetes and yourself—is a matter of life and death.

CHAPTER 3

Diabetes Complications and Long-Term Concerns

It can be hard to face each day knowing you have to test your blood glucose, watch what you eat, keep records, and all the rest. But keeping tight control and taking care of yourself now can help you keep the dreaded long-term complications of diabetes at bay.

The Bad News—*and* the Good

People with diabetes are vulnerable to a variety of problems that develop after they have had the disease for many years. A person with diabetes is more likely than other people to have a heart attack, a stroke, eye problems that can lead to blindness, kidney disease, a foot or leg amputation, frequent infections, and sexual problems. All of these are truly serious long-term problems and are more likely to occur if blood glucose levels have been high over many years.

Fortunately, in this new century, diabetes complications and other problems are no longer inevitable—unless you and your team do not take good care now. People with diabetes can live long, healthful, and productive lives. To do so challenges you and your health care team to become intimately involved in recognizing, treating, and doing whatever it takes to prevent or delay the long-term problems of diabetes.

There are three key areas that will help you to treat, delay, or, better yet, prevent diabetes complications. You need to start with education. Learn the how, what, and why of complications. While these problems may be scary to think about, learning about them can help you to take a proactive stance. Next, understand the earliest signs and symptoms of problems. Know your lab test results and keep track of changes. Any change, even when results are normal, may indicate that problems might be starting to develop.

Fighting Complications

There are three keys to treating, delaying, or preventing diabetes complications:

Education	Learn as much as you can about diabetes.
Early Detection	Learn the signs and symptoms of potential problems.
Regular Office Visits	Set up a schedule, and *stick to it!*

Finally, make regular office visits with your health care team and keep the appointments, even if you are feeling well. See your team at least every three months when you are doing and feeling well, and contact them immediately if you are having problems. Working together, you and your health professionals will form a strong prevention team.

How Do Problems Start?

When blood glucose levels exceed 140 mg/dl, the glucose becomes toxic to your body. The excess glucose spills over into the urine causing frequent urination and, consequently, increased thirst. This leads to dehydration, which causes muscle cramps and dizziness. Because the glucose is not getting into the cells very well, if at all, your cells can't get the energy they need to function. You feel fatigued and hungry and you may begin to lose weight. In addition, the excess glucose impairs the ability of your white blood cells to fight off infections and heal wounds. Finally, your vision becomes blurry and you experience great fluctuations in your sight. This occurs because glucose has entered the lenses of your eyes. Inside your lenses, the glucose is changed to sorbitol. The sorbitol pulls water into the lenses, which causes them to swell. This swelling changes the shape of your lenses, and this affects your sight.

These changes in your body are generally recognized as the "early warning signs" of diabetes, and one or more of these may even have sent you to your doctor in the first place. All of these problems are completely reversible with the normalization of your glucose levels. It is only when your body is bathed in toxic glucose levels over time that these problems continue and the long-term complications of diabetes develop.

Why Do Problems Continue?

There are two significant events that take place when glucose remains above 140 mg/dl over extended periods of time. The first event is the formation of *advanced glycated end products*, also known as AGEs, and the second event is *oxidation*.

Have you ever looked at a freshly baked turkey and noticed how the skin has turned a golden brown and become stiff and crispy? Well, that is an example of glucose combining with protein, in an oven at 350 degrees Fahrenheit, to form advanced glycated end products. In the human body, glucose combines with protein in the same way but is baked at the lower temperature of 98.6 degrees Fahrenheit. The development of these long-lived products occurs in everyone and accumulates with aging. For people with diabetes, who have elevated glucose levels, these AGEs form at an accelerated rate. As the AGEs accumulate, the proteins in your body thicken, become brittle, and no longer slip and slide as well. This is the cause of some of the shoulder pain and stiffness of the joints in people who have poorly controlled diabetes. More seriously, the accumulation of AGEs affects the blood vessels of the kidneys, eyes, feet, and large blood vessels of the body, causing complications.

The other event that occurs at an accelerated rate in diabetes is *oxidation*. Oxidation is the process that causes rust on cars. Similar damage occurs naturally in the human body. When your body breaks down glucose for energy, by-products called free radicals are made. These free radicals add oxygen to everything in sight, damaging cellular tissue. It is as if your bloodstream and blood vessels are rusting out. As this "rusting" continues, it damages the linings of your blood vessels and causes various tissues in your body to malfunction. If glucose levels are elevated, high numbers of free radicals are formed and more "rusting," or oxidation, occurs.

Seeing After Your Eyes

Ever wonder how your eyes see? You see an object when light is reflected off of it and directed back to your eye. The light enters your eye through a clear covering called the cornea. It passes through the lens, which focuses the light onto the retina, the light-sensing tissue at the back of the eye. The retina translates these visual signals into electrical impulses that are sent, by way of the optic nerve, to the brain so that we can see the image. The retina is supplied with nutrients and oxygen by a network of very small blood vessels. If glucose levels are elevated, AGEs and oxidation cause the small blood vessels in the retina to thicken in some parts and weaken in others. This leads to the development of diabetic retinopathy, a disease of the small blood vessels of the retina of the eye.

Danger Signs

You may not have any signs of retina damage from your diabetes. But if you experience one or more of the following symptoms, see your eye doctor:

- Blurry or double vision

- Rings, flashing lights, or blank spots

- Dark or floating spots

- Pain or pressure in one or both of your eyes

- Trouble seeing things out of the corners of your eyes

As the tiny blood vessels in the retina become swollen, they leak a little fluid into the center of the retina, which may cause your sight to become permanently blurred. This condition is called *background retinopathy*. If the retinopathy progresses, the deterioration of your sight will progress as well. To try to supply the retina with nutrients and oxygen, many new, tiny blood vessels grow across the eye. This is called *neovascularization*. These vessels are very fragile and break easily, causing bleeding into the center of your eye, blocking vision and causing blindness.

Modern Eyes

Laser technology can now be used in the early stages of retinopathy to stop the bleeding from the fragile blood vessels in the eyes.

Scar tissue may also form near the retina, pulling it away from the back of the eye. This stage is called *proliferative retinopathy*, and it can lead to impaired vision and even blindness.

Treatment for diabetic retinopathy can help prevent loss of vision and can sometimes restore some lost vision or stop the progression of neovascularization. Thanks to modern medicine and the invention and application of laser technology, neovascularization can be treated. A laser beam can be focused on these excessive and fragile blood vessels, causing them to clot and stop bleeding. But this has to be done early in the course of the disease to be effective.

While research is progressing to alter blood flow in the eyes to prevent the early changes of diabetic retinopathy, the best form of treatment is preven-

Get Checked

Sound medical management of your diabetes by you and your team and regular eye exams can all but eliminate diabetic retinopathy.

tion. It is now well known that there are two essential things you can do to best safeguard your vision: Control your blood glucose levels and have regularly scheduled eye exams. Sound medical management of your diabetes by you and your team and regular, yearly eye examinations can all but eliminate retinopathy. In addition, for 95 percent of people with diabetes who are already affected by some abnormal blood-vessel growth, early screening and prompt treatment can prevent blindness.

In addition to retinopathy, people with diabetes can have other eye problems that demand atten- tion. *Glaucoma*, which is caused by too much pressure in the eye, can occur in anyone and is a problem that is not related to diabetes. However, people with diabetes have a greater risk of developing glaucoma. You may have no symptoms of glaucoma, but it can be diagnosed with a simple test that measures pressure in your eye. If detected, it should be treated promptly. When glaucoma is undetected or left untreated, blindness results, which is yet another reason to have regular eye exams by an eye doctor. Treatment for glaucoma is usually simple and consists of using special eyedrops to lower the pressure in your eye. Eye doctors sometimes recommend laser surgery.

Another common eye problem is *cataracts*, a condition in which the lens of the eye becomes cloudy. This happens in a lot of people as they get older; however, cataracts are more common in people with diabetes. The cloudy crystals in the lens of the eye are caused in part by AGEs. They can lead to poor night vision and, eventually, blindness if not treated. They are treated by removing the lens and replacing it with an implant. Such surgery is done routinely without complications at surgical centers, and most patients are right back to their usual routine within a day or two.

The latest techniques in modern medicine can indeed help to prevent blindness caused by diabetes. But the key is to catch changes early. And that's why regular screening is essential.

Keeping Your Kidneys Fit

Your kidneys have many functions, but the most important are getting rid of products from your blood by excreting them in urine and maintaining a proper mineral and fluid balance in your body. In this way, your kidneys are a bit like a filter or sieve, keeping the right amounts of the good stuff in and getting rid of what you don't need.

There are a tremendous number of tiny blood vessels that feed the very small cavities in your kidneys, much like the many tiny blood vessels that feed the tissues in your eyes. The vessels in the kidneys have selective-size pores that allow certain molecules to fall into the cavities and be carried out with the urine while at the same time

How Do I Take Care of My Kidneys?

Have a screening test done yearly for microalbumin.

Improve your blood glucose control.

Maintain a normal blood pressure.

Avoid medications that can be damaging to your kidneys.

Avoid all forms of nicotine.

Use preventive medications, ACE inhibitors, when needed.

Lower your intake of protein.

preventing needed molecules from leaving the body. When your glucose levels remain elevated, AGEs build up in the wall of the blood vessels, causing the vessels to become abnormally porous. In addition to AGEs, high blood pressure, nicotine, and certain other conditions can damage the small blood vessels of the kidney. As a result, protein molecules start leaking through the pores in the vessels.

In the early stages of kidney disease, *albumin*, the major protein in your blood, begins to leak through the damaged vessels at an abnormal rate. This condition is called *proteinuria*, or in the earliest stages, *microalbuminuria*, since only small amounts of protein appear in the urine. Normally, less than 30 micrograms (a microgram, mcg, is one millionth of a gram) of albumin are found in your urine on any given day. Results that are greater than 30 micrograms are confirmed by a repeat test, and if positive, indicate that damage has occurred to your kidney's blood vessels.

As the kidney disease progresses, the pores in the kidney's vessels become larger due to the damage, and more protein is lost. When the protein loss reaches 1,000 milligrams, or 1 gram, each day, you may notice puffiness in your ankles due to fluid buildup (edema). The waste products slowly begin to collect in the blood (this buildup can be measured and is called your *serum creatinine level*), as the kidneys become less effective at filtering. As the creatinine level increases, so do the levels of other waste products, causing you to become nauseated and fatigued. The waste buildup poisons the kidneys, harming their ability to make erythropoietin, a substance needed by your bone marrow to make oxygen-carrying red blood cells; you become anemic, which means your body's cells become starved for oxygen. At this point, your kidneys can no longer do their most

> ### Remember!
>
> Maintaining the health of your kidneys starts with a yearly screening test for the presence of micro-albumin in your urine.

basic job, and you require dialysis. Dialysis involves being hooked to a machine that removes the wastes from your blood.

But kidney disease and the slow deterioration of your body's filtering system does not need to happen. There are several ways you can protect your kidneys and reduce the likelihood of kidney problems, prevent current problems from becoming worse, and even reverse problems that have started.

Maintaining the health of your kidneys starts with a yearly screening for microalbumin. This is a very specific test that looks for small amounts of protein in the urine that cannot be detected by the usual "dipstick" test done during a routine urinalysis. It is, however, important to know that an infection, severe stress, heart failure, or strenuous exercise before a screening test can also cause increased levels of protein in your urine. You should have a positive screening test confirmed with a full 24-hour microalbumin test. If the second test is positive, you should then be started on treatment that will return this number to normal.

To keep your kidneys healthy or prevent problems from becoming worse, you need to improve your blood glucose control. Kidney problems result from the increased glucose load, causing a buildup of AGEs. The closer to normal you keep your blood glucose levels, the better for your kidneys. With the guidance of your team, strive for an HbA1c (which will be discussed more thoroughly in Chapter 6) of less than seven percent, or even less than six percent if that's possible without risking hypoglycemia (low blood glucose).

Make sure you maintain a normal blood pressure. When blood pressure is above 130/85 mm Hg, it slowly damages your kidneys. Have your blood pressure checked often, and learn how to monitor it yourself at home. If it is consistently high, early treatment is important. Nicotine, salt, caffeine, and alcohol all can raise blood pressure. By contrast, adding some physical activity and extra movement to your life can help lower your blood pressure.

Make sure you avoid medications that can be damaging to the kidneys. When your doctor chooses a drug, such as an antibiotic to treat an infection, confirm that kidney damage is not a possible side effect. Be aware that some over-the-counter drugs can cause problems as well. Excessive use of nonsteroidal anti-inflammatory drugs (NSAIDs), such as aspirin, ibuprofen, and naproxen, can cause kidney damage. It is safe to use these as recommended on the bottle once in a while. But large daily doses have been associated with kidney problems, so if you have ongoing pain or inflammation, talk to your doctor before self-medicating with large doses of NSAIDs.

To maintain the health of your kidneys, you must avoid all forms of nicotine. Nicotine is as harmful to the kidneys as untreated high blood pressure is. Because nicotine is so addictive, the best policy is never to start smoking. If you already smoke or chew tobacco, talk to your doctor about programs or medications that can help you to stop—soon!

To help slow or reverse kidney disease, it is recommended that prescription medications called *angiotensin-converting enzyme (ACE) inhibitors* be used when needed. Studies have shown that this class of blood pressure medicines can slow kidney disease and protect the kidneys from further damage. In addition, ACE inhibitors also prevent damage to other blood vessels in the body. Started slowly and taken until there is a change in your kidney status, they will not abnormally lower your blood pressure. And if you are currently taking a medication for high blood pressure, speak with your doctor and make sure you are on an ACE inhibitor.

Finally, lower the amount of protein in your diet, since it can aggravate kidney problems. When your kidney function begins to decrease, it generally helps to slow down the process by eating less protein. The protein is an extra load for the kidneys to handle, as the nitrogen from the breakdown of proteins tends to poison the kidneys. For an exact dietary prescription to maintain your kidney health, consult your doctor, diabetes educator, and dietitian.

Taking Care of Your Tootsies

Diabetes is the most common cause of limb loss, other than accidents, in the United States. Problems begin in your legs or your feet due to changes in your blood vessels and nerves; those changes are caused by excess glucose, AGEs, and oxidation. Blood vessels become blocked, and your legs and feet do not receive enough blood. This causes aching pains in your legs and feet, especially when walking, and sores that heal slowly.

To compound the problem, your nerves become poisoned by the high levels of glucose, resulting in pain, numbness, and a tingling feeling in your feet and legs, all of which dull the sensitivity of your nerves and your ability to sense a potential problem with your feet. You may not notice a sore caused by a tight, rubbing shoe or a blister from a new pair of shoes. If ignored and left untreated, the sore can become infected and, due to poor blood circulation, may possibly lead to the need for amputation of the affected area.

Feet First

You can prevent foot problems that lead to amputation with careful attention to foot health and regular visits with your health care team.

Amputations never need to happen. Proper foot care and regular visits to your health care team can prevent foot and leg sores and ensure that any that do appear don't become infected and painful. Foot care is a combined effort by you and your doctor. You need to know what you can do to prevent problems and what to expect from your doctor as well.

Self-care includes the inspection of your feet for sores, cuts, or infection. Get a handheld mirror and examine your feet thoroughly every day. Clean your feet daily and dry them well, especially between the toes, and keep them soft by using lotion after a bath or shower. When you buy shoes, have both the width and length of each foot measured to make sure your shoes fit well and have enough space for your toes. Never go barefoot, even in the home, where you can accidentally kick furniture or step on something sharp hidden in the carpeting. If you go to the beach, wear sandals or water socks to protect your feet from sharp objects and pointy rocks in the sand. And finally, never, ever, do "bathroom surgery" on your feet. Corns, calluses, ingrown toenails, and thick, fungal nails are best left to a podiatrist, or foot doctor. A podiatrist can do foot surgery, trim your nails, and prescribe medications for your feet when needed. You need to see a podiatrist regularly if you have lost any sensation in your feet, if you cannot cut your own nails, or if you have an ulcer on your foot.

It is also your responsibility to assist your health care team in the care of your feet by being prepared for your team visit. Uncover your feet before the doctor enters the room; wear shoes and socks that make this easy to do. Tell your doctor about any foot-care concerns or questions. Have the doctor inspect all surfaces of your feet, including the soles and between the toes. Make sure your doctor checks the pulses in your feet, as well. This lets you both know how well the blood is circulating to your feet. Finally, your doctor should do a special test to check the sensation in your feet. If the results show that you have lost the protective sensation in your feet, you are vulnerable to infections, sores, and ultimately, foot loss. This problem alone, or in combination with limited circulation, can potentially spell real trouble. It means you need to take extra precautions to keep your feet safe. And while you cannot always avoid a loss of sensation or decreased circulation in your legs, studies have shown that you have a better chance of avoiding these problems if you take good care of your feet, do not smoke, and keep both your blood pressure and diabetes under good control.

CHAPTER 4

Diabetes and Syndrome X

If you have Type 2 diabetes, you more than likely also have the mysterious-sounding Syndrome X. The two can be a deadly combination unless you take steps to monitor them regularly and keep them both under control.

The Discovery

In the mid-1970s, Dr. Gerald Reaven at Stanford University Medical Center described a condition that he coined "Syndrome X." He noted a clustering of medical conditions that were associated with a very high rate of coronary artery disease (a common type of heart disease that affects the blood vessels feeding the heart). These conditions included high blood pressure, glucose intolerance, and abnormal levels of cholesterol and triglycerides and were associated with insulin resistance and, consequently, high insulin levels. Since the discovery of Syndrome X, there has been a great deal of focus and many studies conducted to try to understand what causes this condition. Some of the resulting fingers of blame point to our ever-expanding waistlines.

The Belly Connection

Each of us is here today because our ancestors had the genetics that allowed them to survive during times of frequent famine and starvation. Back then, if you had a fast metabolism, required a lot of food to maintain your weight, and lost weight readily when food was scarce, you didn't survive. Those that did survive the lean times passed on their genes, and that inheritance is still apparent today. These "thrifty" genes are still bent on helping us conserve calories and are reluctant to let us lose fat stores.

For those of us who live in this land of plenty—a land that's thankfully short on famine but also short on manual labor—these same genes make it difficult to lose extra weight. To compound this effect, if you weighed less than six pounds when you were born, your body chemistry tends to favor conserving fat. And, of course, there's no ignoring the fact that here in America, the older we get, the less active we tend to become, which means our fat stores just keep piling up. In people whose fat stores accumulate primarily in the abdominal area, as opposed to the hips and thighs, an ever-expanding waistline sets the stage for Syndrome X.

Where the Food Goes

When you eat, your food is broken down in your small intestines into three basic nutrients—amino acids, glucose, and fatty acids. From your intestines, the nutrients enter the bloodstream, where they can be picked up and used by the cells that need them.

The cells pluck amino acids from the bloodstream and use them to build a wide array of necessary proteins. In a pinch, the amino acids can also be broken down for energy; some can even be made into glucose. But because of protein's many other important and unique roles, the body generally uses amino acids for energy only when it cannot get enough from carbohydrate and fat. The body

---

The Food You Eat Is Made of:

PROTEINS **CARBOHYDRATES** **FATS**

which are then broken down in your gut into:

AMINO ACIDS **GLUCOSE** **FATTY ACIDS**

which are then used by the body's cells for basic functions, burned for energy, or, when we take in more energy than we need, stored as:

PROTEIN **GLYCOGEN** **TRIGLYCERIDES**

(primarily as part of muscle tissue) | (in the muscles) | (in fat cells deep in your abdomen or in surface fat cells found all over the body) does not have a storage form of amino acids; if too many are taken in, it will break them down, excrete parts of them, and turn the remnants over to be stored as glucose or fatty acids. So when other fuels are not available and the body is forced to call upon amino acids for energy, the body must divert them from their other uses or break down protein that is already in use elsewhere (such as in muscle tissue).

The glucose molecules released from the intestines go to the liver and to the cells, where they can be immediately broken down for energy or stored in the form of glycogen. The muscle cells take in the greatest amount of glucose, which they tend to keep for themselves. The liver also maintains a store of glycogen, which it breaks down into glucose and shares with the brain and other tissues between meals. Glucose is a readily available form of fuel for the cells, but because glucose molecules hold a lot of water and are therefore rather large, the body can only store a limited amount of them.

The fatty acids from a meal also enter the bloodstream and head toward the liver, where they can be picked and used or stored for energy. The liver packages the fatty acids and sends them out to be used by the cells or stored in the form of triglycerides. These dense packets of fat are the body's main form of stored energy. Triglycerides are stored in two primary places: inside the fat cells that are deep in your abdomen, called intra-abdominal fat, and in the surface fat cells found all over your body. While the body needs some fat stores, trouble begins when far too much energy is taken in compared to the amounts expended.

The Battle Ensues

When you continuously take in extra energy, more and more fatty acids are stored as triglycerides. As a result, the fat cells become larger and larger until they reach a limit where no more fatty acids can enter the cells. The fat cells, in an attempt to keep out any more fatty acids, develop a resist-ance to insulin, the hormone trying to force more fatty acids into these cells. When this resistance occurs, the fatty acids begin to build up in the blood. In an attempt to overcome the insulin resistance, your pancreas responds by making more insulin. Not to be one-upped, the fat cells increase their resistance to insulin again.

As a result of this battle, you now have increased amounts of free fatty acids *and* increased levels of insulin in your bloodstream. That's bad news, because the fatty acids head back to your liver, where some are turned into triglycerides and stored in the liver, causing a "fatty liver." The excess fatty acids also begin to irritate the liver, causing your liver enzymes to increase as well. As a response, just like your fat cells, your liver cells put up a wall of resistance to the insulin that is now trying to push the fatty acids inside. Now your liver has become resistant to insulin, and again your pancreas tries to overcome the resistance by making even more insulin. Fighting back, the liver resistance increases, multiplying further the amounts of free fatty acids and circulating insulin in your body.

> ### All Full
>
> When your fat cells become resistant to the effects of insulin, excess amounts of free fatty acids and insulin build up in your bloodstream.

Things go downhill from there. Remember that your body gets glucose from two sources: from the food you eat and, when you are in a fasting state, from your liver. Insulin is responsible for controlling the glucose release from the liver. When the liver can detect the insulin, it does not release glucose. But when insulin levels are low, indicating a fasting state, your liver steps up its release of glucose.

When your liver puts up the walls of resistance to keep out the fatty acids, it can no longer detect the insulin in the blood, so it starts to pour out extra glucose, and blood glucose levels start to rise. To try to combat this increase in glucose, your ever-alert pancreas pours out even more insulin, further adding to the already increasing amounts of circulating insulin.

With the liver satisfactorily keeping out the fatty acids, the fatty acids search out a new home—and they find your muscles. Unlike your glucose-dependent brain, your muscles can use either glucose or fatty acids for energy. Because fatty acids are now very abundant and are so easy to use, your muscles switch to using the fatty acids for fuel (sort of like kids who, given the choice, would rather eat their dessert than their vegetables!). In doing so, your muscles block the incoming glucose. They do this by building up a resistance to the insulin that is trying to push the glucose into the muscle cells. Since your muscles are normally responsible for taking up more than 80 percent of the glucose in your blood, their switch to using fatty acids has a profound effect on your blood glucose levels. As your blood glucose levels slowly start to increase above normal, you become what is called glucose intolerant—your tissues resist taking in glucose despite the presence of large amounts of insulin.

As the blood glucose levels continue to rise, your pancreas tries in vain to lower those levels by further increasing insulin production, and your circulating

insulin levels rise again. You've now entered an endless loop, with ever-increasing levels of circulating insulin, free fatty acids, and glucose, which now start to become toxic to your system.

Toxic: What Do You Mean "Toxic"?

Let's start with the fatty acids. Since the excess fatty acids cannot be made into energy by the liver, they are made into triglycerides and released into your bloodstream. In order to make these triglycerides, your body must rob parts from other fat molecules, most specifically, from your cholesterol molecules.

One of the two main types of cholesterol molecules in your body is the high-density lipoprotein, or HDL, cholesterol. It is often called the "good" cholesterol because it removes fatty acids from your arteries so they can be eliminated from the body. The other type of cholesterol molecule is the low-density lipoprotein, or LDL, cholesterol. LDL cholesterol is often referred to as "bad" cholesterol because it tends to deposit fat in the walls of your arteries.

Unfortunately, it's the beneficial HDL molecules that take the biggest hit when the liver scavenges for parts in order to make triglycerides; the HDL level in the blood drops as a result. Parts of your LDL molecules are also used in the making of triglycerides; the effect, however, is not fewer LDL molecules but simply smaller ones. These small LDL molecules are too small to be picked out of the blood by the liver, so they don't get cleared out of the body. Instead, they continue to circulate in your blood, which allows them plenty of time to find a nice, cozy weak spot on your artery walls where they can attach themselves. What you end up with, then, are high triglyceride levels, low levels of the beneficial HDL cholesterol, and a lot of small, artery-clogging LDL cholesterol molecules in your blood—all of which spell t-r-o-u-b-l-e for your arteries.

If that's not bad enough, you still have all that extra insulin circulating through your blood, and it's doing a number on your blood pressure. The high insulin levels caused by insulin resistance drive the blood pressure up above normal, although exactly how is unclear. The excess of insulin may result in a continuous overstimulation of the blood vessels, causing them to constrict and forcing the blood pressure above normal. In addition, the high insulin levels cause your kidneys to retain more salt, and therefore more water, which increases your blood volume; the extra blood volume, in turn, exerts greater pressure on the walls of your blood vessels.

Your high insulin levels also cause the inside lining of your blood vessels to overproduce a substance called PAI-1 (pronounced "pie one"). PAI-1 is the main contributor to the clotting of your blood. When PAI-1 levels are high, your blood clots more readily, which increases the risk of heart attacks and strokes. To make matters worse, the platelets, the tiny cells in the blood that contribute to clotting, become sticky and form clots more readily as well.

During this whole process, the elevated amounts of glucose in your blood start their slow, destructive process, even though the blood glucose levels may not yet have risen into the diabetic range. As discussed in the previous chapter, free radicals and AGEs begin to accumulate, affecting the tiny blood vessels of the kidneys, eyes, and feet and the large blood vessels throughout the body. Gradually, various tissues throughout your body stop functioning properly.

Do I Have Syndrome X?

The answer is most likely a yes. More than 90 percent of people with Type 2 diabetes have Syndrome X. There is no one test that confirms the diagnosis, but there are symptoms as well as laboratory tests that indicate the presence of this syndrome. If you have one or more of the following signs in addition to having Type 2 diabetes, then you may have Syndrome X.

CENTRAL OBESITY Central obesity refers specifically to the type of obesity that is marked by excess fat in the abdominal area as opposed to fat in the buttocks and thighs. This type of obesity more commonly occurs in men and in postmenopausal women.

HIGH BLOOD PRESSURE (HYPERTENSION) High blood pressure may be caused by the increased levels of circulating insulin, as discussed earlier. It is estimated that Syndrome X is responsible for the high blood pressure in half of all obese people.

DYSLIPIDEMIA Dyslipidemia means high levels of triglycerides, low levels of HDL cholesterol, and small LDL cholesterol molecules.

ANGINA AND HEART ATTACKS Angina (the chest pain caused by narrowing of the arteries leading to the heart) and heart attacks are caused by Syndrome X in more than half of all patients seen in the hospital setting.

FAMILY HISTORY OF TYPE 2 DIABETES The majority of people who have Syndrome X have a family history of Type 2 diabetes. There may also be a family history of coronary artery disease.

ACANTHOSIS NIGRICANS Acanthosis nigricans is a skin condition that causes a darkening and thickening of the skin of your neck and the body folds such as the armpits, the groin area, and the area underneath your breasts. The elevated levels of insulin in your body stimulate the growth of skin in these areas, and the resulting skin is darker and thicker.

POLYCYSTIC OVARY SYNDROME (PCOS) This is another condition that appears to be caused by the high levels of insulin. PCOS is characterized by infertility, lack of menstrual periods, and obesity. Just as with acanthosis nigricans, it is caused by the elevated insulin levels stimulating a portion of the ovaries to overproduce male hormones, which throw off the menstrual cycle and cause acne and increased hair growth.

How Is Syndrome X Related to Diabetes?

That is a good question, and we as yet do not have a complete answer. Obviously, the continued demand on the beta cells of the pancreas to produce insulin puts a strain on these cells. There may also be some toxic by-product of excess insulin secretion that accumulates in the beta cells. The buildup of fatty acids and the increasing glucose levels may slowly poison the beta cells. And finally, it is believed that your genes may also play some unknown role.

In any case, with increasing age, weight, and inactivity, the resistance to insulin increases, leading to higher and higher levels of insulin, free fatty acids, and glucose. During this "silent" period, your body is exposed to these toxins, causing hypertension and dyslipidemia. In 20 percent of the people who have Syndrome X, the beta cells slowly lose the ability to make insulin, and the first sign of diabetes to appear is the abnormal increase of the blood glucose level after a meal. At this stage, diabetes is usually only detected by an oral glucose tolerance test. If not diagnosed at this time, within two or three years the elevated levels of glucose and free fatty acids lead to the further loss of insulin secretion by your pancreas. Your pancreas just plain begins to poop out, overwhelmed by the demand for insulin to manage the ever increasing levels of glucose. The increase in glucose levels now occurs even in the fasting state, right when you get up in the morning and before meals. Once your fasting glucose levels are more than 180 mg/dl, the symptoms of diabetes usually appear, sending you to the doctor. At this point, it is likely that you have already had Syndrome X for more than ten years!

A One-Two Punch to Your Arteries

The combination of Syndrome X and diabetes causes the blood vessel disease atherosclerosis, or hardening of the arteries. Cholesterol builds up in your artery walls because you have too much LDL cholesterol and too little HDL cholesterol to take it away. The LDL cholesterol becomes oxidized, which makes it more irritating to the artery and leads to a local inflammation of the artery wall. This irritation, as well as the accumulation of fat from the LDL molecules, weakens the wall of the artery. The wall eventually cracks, causing an irregularity in the smooth lining of the blood vessel. Your blood's platelets and clotting factors see this wound and attach to it, which leads to a sudden obstruction of one of your blood vessels.

If the obstruction, or clot, occurs in the arteries around your heart, it causes a sudden heart attack. If it develops more slowly, you are likely to experience angina, which is chest discomfort that is brought on by exertion and relieved by rest.

If the clot occurs in the arteries to the brain (cerebral arteries), you will experience either a transient ischemic attack (TIA), which occurs when the obstruction clears quickly, or a stroke. In either case, the symptoms are a sudden onset of one-sided blindness, weakness or numbness, or an inability to speak.

If the obstruction of a vessel occurs in the arteries of your kidney, you will feel nothing. However, your blood creatinine level, which is used to gauge kidney function, will gradually rise. This indicates that damage has been done. If this same type of obstruction suddenly occurs in the artery to your leg, you will develop severe leg pain and the leg will become cold. Many times, the obstruction of the leg artery occurs slowly; this is called claudication. The symptoms of claudication are calf or hip pain on exertion that is relieved by rest. If you are not active, the only symptoms of claudication may be red or purple toes whenever you dangle your feet, loss of hair on your lower legs, thinning of the skin on your feet, or a foot ulcer.

Most people with Syndrome X and diabetes have atherosclerosis. For this reason, it is of great importance that you prevent and/or detect and treat these conditions. Very often, the symptoms of possible heart problems may be vague, or they may not occur at all. If you do experience any discomfort in your chest, you should contact your doctor. A screening EKG, a painless test that measures electrical signals coming from your heart, can be done to detect a problem. Although an important tool, the EKG is not very sensitive or specific, so you may need to take an exercise stress test (in which your heart function is monitored as you walk on a treadmill). Depending on your risk factors and symptoms, your doctor may also order an angiogram, in which dye is injected into the blood vessels to visualize any narrowing or blockage.

Likewise, if you experience any symptoms of sudden and transient vision loss in one eye or temporary weakness in one side or the other, contact your doctor at once. Your doctor can listen to the sounds of your blood flowing through the arteries in your neck (called the carotid arteries) to detect narrowing in these blood vessels. The doctor can then order tests of the carotid arteries to spot any obstructions.

Butt Out!

If you're a smoker, quitting nicotine can bring great improvements in your health. When you stop smoking or chewing tobacco, you improve the health of your blood vessels. Quitting also means your skin won't age as quickly and you'll be less likely to suffer lung disease and cancer. And there's an additional benefit if you're a man: If you quit smoking, you'll be less likely to suffer impotence.

If you smoke or chew tobacco, get advice from your health care team about how to quit. Your local hospital or the local chapter of the American Cancer Society or the American Lung Association (see Resources) can also provide advice and link you with support groups.

You might also want to consider medication to help you quit, especially if you smoke more than a pack a day. Nicotine replacement now comes in patches, gum, and inhalers. Even though the nicotine in these products is still dangerous, it's not nearly as dangerous as the episodic high levels of nicotine and other toxic chemicals your body is exposed to when you smoke.

Zyban, a recently introduced prescription antidepressant that acts on the addiction centers of the brain, may also help you. It can help minimize the cravings that are associated with quitting smoking. Talk to your doctor and find out if this medication is right for you.

Also, if you notice any symptoms of claudication, report them to your doctor so that the appropriate tests can be done to detect any blockages.

What Can I Do to Treat Syndrome X?

Increasing your level of activity and changing your relationship with food are great places to start. These changes are usually not expensive and generally quite safe and are the cornerstones of treatment for both Syndrome X and diabetes. For some people, these changes are enough to decrease the levels of insulin resistance and diminish the signs of the syndrome. In addition, there are also medications available for the treatment of the various components of Syndrome X.

LOW-DOSE ASPIRIN An 81 mg aspirin tablet, taken daily, is moderately effective in making the platelets in your blood less "sticky," so they are less likely to attach to rough spots in your arteries. This significantly counteracts the clot-forming tendencies of Syndrome X and can reduce the risk of death from heart disease by more than one-third. If you have asthma, an aspirin allergy, or a bleeding problem, however, you should not take aspirin. In some cases, if you are taking aspirin or aspirinlike medications for chronic pain or arthritis, you may not need to take the low-dose aspirin.

Before you consider taking a daily dose of aspirin, however, be sure to consult your doctor.

STATINS Newer medications, called statins, have made managing dyslipidemia easy. These medications have proven themselves to be very safe and yet powerful in lowering LDL cholesterol. Common statin brand names include Baycol, Lipitor, Loescol, Mevacor, Pravachol, and Zocor.

Statins all work the same way, by reducing the ability of your liver to make LDL cholesterol and by increasing your liver's uptake and destruction of the LDL cholesterol molecules in the blood. In addition, statins raise HDL and lower triglyceride levels, especially when used in high doses. They are usually taken at bedtime and have just a few side effects. Liver irritation occurs in about 1 to 3 of every 1,000 patients treated, but it usually goes away when the medication is stopped. To monitor the liver, a blood test, called ALT, is done 6 to 12 weeks after starting the medication and once a year after that. You may also experience other side effects, such as fatigue, insomnia, depression, headaches, rash, or intestinal upset with these medications, but these side effects are rare.

Even more rare, but potentially fatal, is rhabdomyolysis, which is a rapid muscle tear down in your body. It is characterized by significant muscle aches and weakness all over your body and occurs more commonly when a statin is combined with certain other medications, such as erythromycin, nicotinic acid, or Lopid. It may also occur more often in older patients who have kidney disease. Should you experience any of these symptoms, it is very important to contact your doctor so that a simple diagnostic blood test, called a CPK, can be done.

> ## Lipid Service
>
> Newer medications called statins are now usually the first drugs used in treating unhealthy cholesterol levels in the blood.

The goal in treating your cholesterol is to get your LDL cholesterol lower than 100 mg/dl and to raise your HDL cholesterol over 45 mg/dl if you are a man or over 55 mg/dl if you are a woman. The goal for your triglycerides is less than 200 mg/dl. If your LDL cholesterol is over 100 mg/dl, you should first try a statin and see what effect it has on your LDL, HDL, and triglycerides. If this is unsuccessful and if you also have multiple risk factors for heart disease or you already have heart disease, you may be placed on a fibric acid or nicotinic acid medication.

FIBRIC ACID The fibric acid medications currently available in the United States are Lopid and Tri-

Cor. They work directly on your liver or endothelium to reduce the triglyceride level and raise the HDL level, but unfortunately they have little effect on LDL cholesterol. Lopid appears to cause more stomach upset and has to be taken twice a day compared to the once-a-day dosing of TriCor. TriCor is best taken first thing in the morning. Many doctors combine TriCor and a statin to get better improvements in all lipid levels, although this combination is not recommended because of the risk of muscle damage.

NICOTINIC ACID Also known as niacin, nicotinic acid is the best medicine for raising HDL levels. It is a vitamin, but when used in high doses, it acts as a drug. Such high doses of niacin also commonly cause numerous side effects, including aggravation of peptic ulcers, gout, facial flushing for a few hours after taking the medication, hives, and other skin conditions. In addition, niacin causes an *increase* in insulin resistance, which is one problem that, as a person with diabetes, you are trying to combat.

ANGIOTENSIN-CONVERTING-ENZYME (ACE) INHIBITORS High blood pressure can be even more damaging if you also have diabetes and Syndrome X. The increased pressure in your arteries accelerates coronary and cerebrovascular disease (heart attacks and strokes) but also contributes to the small blood vessel disease in your kidneys and eyes. Your goal is to get your blood pressure as low as possible without side effects, such as dizziness upon standing. And there are many new classes of medications to help you.

ACE inhibitors lower your blood pressure, protect the lining of your blood vessels, and reduce insulin resistance. In several recently reported studies, the incidence of diabetes in people who were at risk for developing the disease was 25 percent less in those receiving ACE inhibitors. Trials are ongoing to study whether ACE inhibitors should be recommended as a preventative in people at high risk for developing diabetes.

A common side effect of ACE inhibitors is a cough. Oddly enough, however, the cough is a good sign. By blocking a certain chemical re-action, ACE inhibitors allow the accumulation of a chemical in the blood that is very protective to the lining of your blood vessels. A cough means that you have this protection. Rare but serious side effects of ACE inhibitors are swelling of the mouth and tongue and an elevation of potassium and creatinine levels in your blood. Blood tests will need to be done periodically to check potassium and creatinine levels.

There are many ACE inhibitors available, including Accupril, Altace, Capoten, Mavik, Monopril, Prinivil, and Vasotec. They are usually taken once a day and are not very expensive.

ANGIOTENSIN BLOCKERS Angiotensin blockers can be substituted for ACE inhibitors in people who cannot tolerate the cough caused by the ACE inhibitors. Angiotensin blockers block chemicals downstream from where the ACE inhibitors work. Although they do not cause a cough, they are more expensive than ACE inhibitors and do not protect the arteries as well. But they can cause increases in potassium and creatinine levels, so treatment with them requires periodic blood testing. Some of the angiotensin blockers available in the United States are Avapro, Cozaar, Diovan, Micardis, and Teveten.

HYDROCHLOROTHIAZIDES Hydrochlorothiazides are diuretics, or "water pills." In both diabetes and Syndrome X, they are used in small doses to reduce blood pressure. In these smaller doses, they appear to lower blood pressure by relaxing the small blood vessels rather than through a diuretic action. In larger doses (above 12.5 mg per day), hydrochlorothiazides cause an increase in insulin resistance and a reduction in insulin secretion by the pancreas. Other side effects, again generally found in doses over 12.5 mg per day, include loss of potassium, rashes, and cramps. There are literally hundreds of brands of hydrochlorothiazides. They are very inexpensive and are taken just once a day, in the morning.

CALCIUM CHANNEL BLOCKERS There are several groups of compounds that block the calcium channels in your artery muscles, causing them to relax. Of the several groups available, the "vasodilating" ones are the best for diabetes because they have the fewest side effects. These drugs include Norvasc and Plendil. They are moderately expensive and have several side effects, including edema and constipation, but they don't increase insulin resistance.

BETA BLOCKERS The beta blockers—including Inderal, Tenormin, and Toprol—are a relatively older group of medications that have both benefits and drawbacks. Studies have shown beta blockers to be especially effective in treating people who have coronary disease, as they have been shown to reduce the chance of dying for people with this condition. In addition, a large study conducted in England and reported in 1998 showed that Tenormin was as good as the ACE inhibitor Capoten in reducing large and small blood vessel disease in people with diabetes. The downside is that the beta blockers cause a variety of unpleasant side effects, including nightmares, insomnia, and depression. They also block your ability to sense hypoglycemia, cause your hands to feel cold, and tend to worsen diabetes control and increase insulin resistance.

COREG Other medications to treat high blood pressure have also been introduced, and some have shown great promise, especially for people who have both Syndrome X and diabetes. One standout is Coreg. Coreg has properties of several of the above-mentioned blood-pressure medications in addition to its ability to lower insulin resistance and reduce the oxidation of blood that occurs in Syndrome X. Coreg can, however, cause dizziness, and it is expensive.

COMBINATION MEDICATION Combinations of the above groups of medications are common. For many people, for example, successful blood pressure management occurs only with a combination of medications. In addition, there tend to be fewer side effects when using small doses of several medications rather than a large dose of one medication. Indeed, some pharmaceutical companies have already combined groups of medications, such as Accupril and hydrochlorothiazide, into one pill, making medicating simpler.

What If My Arteries Are Already Narrowed?

Major advances have been made in methods for unplugging heart arteries with balloons and lasers. When a sudden clot occurs, there now are powerful medicines that can be given to dissolve the clot and keep the heart muscle from dying. And surgery to bypass blocked arteries is safer and less traumatic than ever. In fact, you are generally up within a day or two of the surgery and home before the week is out.

In the event of a full stroke, getting to emergency care very quickly can make all the difference. Medication is now available to dissolve a clot in the arteries supplying the brain, but it must be administered within the first few hours of the stroke. New medicines are also being developed to protect the brain or even to restore the brain after a stroke.

Clots in the arteries of the legs can now often be dissolved nonsurgically as well. And new techniques allow surgery to be performed on smaller and smaller arteries.

CHAPTER 5

Monitoring Your Glucose

To achieve glucose levels that are as close to normal as possible, you need to regularly monitor them. Today, the meters available for glucose testing are small, convenient, and relatively easy to use, making monitoring an easier and more effective part of your diabetes care. What's more, the testing methods on the horizon may very well make testing automatic and painless.

From Tasting to Testing

In 400 B.C., ancient Indian physicians noted that people suffering the symptoms of diabetes had a sweet taste to their urine. It would not be until A.D. 1600 that Thomas Willis would rediscover the same sweet taste of diabetic urine. By 1848, the first urine test for glucose was developed, which lead to the early understanding of diabetes. Prior to the development of this test, it was the job of the assistants to the physician to taste the urine of patients to determine a diagnosis of diabetes. Glucose testing back then was truly an unpleasant task!

In 1908, a method for measuring glucose in the blood would be discovered, but it would be confined to the laboratory, for use only by physicians, for the next 60 years. People with diabetes were left with urine testing at home. Urine testing, however, could only detect high glucose levels, and only hours after the blood glucose had been elevated.

In the late 1960s, blood glucose measuring was first introduced for home use, representing one of the most important advances in controlling diabetes since the discovery of insulin in 1921. People with diabetes were able to detect high *and* low blood sugar levels by placing a single drop of blood on a chemical test strip and watching for a color change on the strip.

The late 1970s saw the introduction of a portable meter that was able to "read" the chemical strips. This change represented a new trend in diabetes management and truly brought the person with diabetes forward as an active and vital part of the diabetes management team.

Today, thanks to technology, there are simple, practical systems for monitoring your blood glucose at home or anyplace you go. Self-monitoring of blood glucose allows you to know, with great accuracy, your blood glucose level, so you can adjust your food, medication, or activity level accordingly and with confidence. It means far greater freedom to participate in any activities you choose, and therefore, far greater control over your life.

To Master, You Must Monitor

Blood glucose monitoring is a vital part of the diabetes management process, and frequent self-monitoring is the key to successful diabetes care. By using glucose testing, you get a precise measurement of what your blood glucose level is at the time of the test. The blood glucose values are like clues in a mystery novel. The more clues you have, the greater your understanding of the mystery. Of course, the opposite can be true as well. The less you test, the fewer clues you have and the more your diabetes stays a mystery to both you and your health care team.

Checking your blood glucose level is essential in managing your diabetes because it is a critical factor in making treatment decisions to prevent the potentially devastating effects of diabetes.

Research has shown that the higher the blood glucose is allowed to be over time, the greater the possibility of problems and serious complications that affect many systems of the body. A national study, the Diabetes Control and Complications Trial, has shown that tightly controlling blood glucose levels can prevent, reduce, or even reverse some of the long-term complications and problems associated with diabetes. It was this study that showed that by maintaining your blood glucose level as close to normal as possible, you may reduce your risk of complications involving your eyes, kidneys, and nervous system by up to 60 percent.

Check, Please!

Self-monitoring of blood glucose allows you to adjust your food, medication, or activity level with greater confidence.

Reducing your risk of serious complications depends upon your keeping blood glucose levels as nearly normal as possible. This level of tight glucose control depends on frequent monitoring. Even for the person whose daily routine rarely changes, all kinds of things, like stress, illness, unanticipated activity, alcohol, or medications, can throw off the balanced routine, resulting in unpleasant and sometimes dangerous consequences.

Testing your blood glucose on a regular basis allows you to know the ongoing status of your diabetes and will allow you to learn more about your diabetes and your body. Testing your blood glucose level multiple times each day will give you even more information. This type of regular testing helps you to understand blood glucose patterns that occur when you eat certain foods and take specific medication doses and how these are connected to your level of activity and stressors at home or work. Frequent glucose testing also ensures that you can respond quickly to high or low blood sugar levels with appropriate intervention.

Your monitor records how your personal glucose levels change in response to ordinary events, such as eating, menstruation, stress, and activity. Then, working together with your health care team and through careful trial, you can find out what works best for you—food, exercise, medications, or insulin—to keep your levels as close to normal as possible.

If you choose not to test your blood glucose levels, you cannot know whether your diabetes is really controlled. You never learn the relationship between what and how much you eat and the effect on your blood glucose. The lows that occur, say, after activity will remain a mystery, as will the high blood glucose levels that may be occurring each morning. Only with frequent glucose testing can you monitor your levels and be assured that they are within the normal range. When done properly, and with support and education from your health care team, glucose testing can allow *you* to modify the type of food you eat, vary the amount and time of exercise, and adjust medications.

Why Urine Testing Isn't Good Enough

Why switch to poking your finger with a needle, when urine testing was so helpful for more than 100 years? It's true that for years the urine test strip was the only link for the person with diabetes to their glucose levels and the only way that level could be measured at home. The results were indirect, measuring the spillover of glucose in the urine, and were of only limited use for total diabetes management. But it was better than having no information at all.

Urine testing is no longer recommended for glucose monitoring because such tests don't show what the glucose level is at the moment of the test but rather what the glucose level was several hours before, after the last urination. In addition,

Why Would I Want to Test My Blood Glucose?

- To identify patterns in my blood glucose control.

- To lead a more flexible life.

- To reduce the risk of long-term diabetic complications.

- To understand the impact of food, activity, and medications on my blood glucose.

- To quickly identify either high or low glucose levels and treat the problem appropriately.

- To figure out what may be causing my high or low blood glucose levels.

- So my health care team has to do less guessing when establishing my diabetes treatment plan.

- To determine the effectiveness of my current diabetes treatment plan.

- To identify when changes are needed in my diabetes treatment plan.

- To evaluate changes in my diabetes treatment plan and see if my glucose levels improve.

- Because numbers are information, and with information I can better manage this disease called diabetes.

- To learn, with the help of my team, how to modify my food intake, level of activity, and medications and still maintain healthy glucose levels.

- Because testing allows me to reach a level of freedom, security, and control that would otherwise be impossible.

- To feel good.

- To live healthy and free from diabetes complications.

urine testing does not tell you how high the blood glucose was, and it tells nothing about low blood glucose events. Only tests on the blood can show both low and high blood glucose levels and can be done as the high or low is occurring. It is the only way for you to build an understanding of the effects of your lifestyle and diabetes treatment plan on your glucose levels and the only way to maintain your glucose levels within a healthy range to prevent the longer term complications of diabetes.

The appeal of urine testing, when compared to blood glucose testing, is understandable. Urine testing is easy, painless, and inexpensive, but today experts agree that measuring glucose in the blood is preferred over urine testing. The only time that urine testing is recommended is when testing for urine ketones is necessary. Ketones are a sign that your body has been using stored fat, rather than blood glucose, for fuel because of a lack of available insulin. When there is not enough insulin present to funnel glucose into your cells, your body tries to use stored fat to make fuel available to your cells. Fat in fat cells is broken down into fatty acids, which pass through the liver and form ketones. Ketones are exhaled and excreted in urine. As you will learn in more detail in later chapters, you will need to test your urine for ketones if your blood sugar levels are running high (240 or more) or when you are ill. The presence of ketones can indicate ketoacidosis, a serious and life-threatening emergency.

What Meter Is Best for Me?

Blood glucose monitoring systems are simpler, faster, and more accurate than ever before. Many meters give test results in seconds, and most will store results for later recall. Meters include many features designed to make self-monitoring convenient. Many operate on batteries, are small enough to fit in a purse or shirt pocket, and can be used almost anywhere. Some contain electronic memory, and more-advanced models even have built-in modems for transmitting the test results to your physician. With so many options available, you should look at several models and discuss their advantages and disadvantages with your health care team to see which model best suits your needs.

The meters that are currently available use one of two methods for measuring blood glucose. The *reflectance photometers* measure light reflected from a test strip after it has undergone a chemical reaction. The *electrochemical meters* measure the electric current produced by the blood resting on the tip of the test strip. The photometric meters have been around the longest and have proved to be reliable and accurate. They use a light source with filters and a lens to detect a color change on the strip caused by glucose in the blood. Electrochemical meters use the newest technology currently available. Glucose in the blood causes a reaction on the test strip that produces a tiny electric current, and the meter detects and "reads" the current. All available meters have been tested for accuracy and approved for home use by the U.S. Food and Drug Administration (FDA).

No Sweat!

The latest blood-glucose meters include many features that make self-monitoring faster, easier, and more accurate than ever before.

In addition to the two methods of measuring blood glucose, meters are also calibrated in one of two ways. Your test results are either reported as a *whole-blood reading* or are *plasma calibrated*. Whole-blood meters measure the glucose present in a drop of whole blood. Plasma-calibrated meters measure the glucose present in a drop of whole blood but then automatically add 12 percent to the measured value. This plasma-calibrated value is equal to the reading that a laboratory might obtain, since all laboratory equipment is set up to measure the glucose that is present in a plasma sample of blood. (A plasma sample is the portion of the blood that remains once the red blood cells are removed.) One type of reading is not better than the other. They both measure your blood glucose. You just need to know how your meter is calibrated so you and your team can set appropriate goals and you can correctly determine the accuracy of your meter when comparing it to a laboratory test result.

When narrowing your choice of meters, and in order to get the most benefit from your monitoring, you should pick the meter that is easiest for you to use and maintain properly. This is crucial because your ability to accurately perform the procedure is an important factor in determining which meter is appropriate and will provide reliable and accurate results.

Meters themselves are usually relatively inexpensive. Many machines are actually available for free at pharmacies and clinics through special offers from manufacturers. Some manufacturers give you a meter free with the purchase of 100 test strips. Most manufacturers of meters offer mail-in rebates after you buy the meter and trade-in rebates if you mail them back your old meter.

This way, if you don't like your original purchase, you can always trade it in for another at little cost. It is important to keep in mind, however, that you should never trade in your current meter based solely on the fact that the new one is free. Check to see if the meter has all the features you feel are important and also check with your health care team to see if the trade would be a "good deal" for you.

If you have insurance, check with your provider regarding the coverage of diabetes supplies and which meter and supplies, if specified, are covered. If you have Medicare, new regulations in effect since

Such a Deal!

Most blood-glucose meters are relatively inexpensive, and some are actually provided free with the purchase of 100 test strips.

July 1998 specify that Medicare will cover the costs of blood testing supplies for people with diabetes. Check with your local Medicare provider for details.

There are currently 9 companies that offer 30 different meters in the United States alone. Your choice of meter will depend, at least in part, on the individual features of the meters. Use the checklist on page 91 to help you narrow your search and select the best meter for you. Simply

What Meter Features Do You Require?

REQUIRED?

YES	NO	Does the speed of testing make a difference? (Meters can take from 6 seconds to 2 minutes to provide results.)
YES	NO	Do you want a meter that "beeps" to prompt you?
YES	NO	Do you want a silent meter?
YES	NO	Is the meter simple to use? (How many steps are there?)
YES	NO	Do you prefer individually wrapped test strips? (Some find the foil-wrapped strips difficult to open, but they are less likely to spoil in high humidity.)
YES	NO	Is the calibration test easy to perform?
YES	NO	Does the meter need to be cleaned? If so, is it easy to do?
YES	NO	Do you need a meter with a memory?
YES	NO	Do you want the meter memory to give you the date and time of the glucose test in addition to the test result?
YES	NO	Do you want the meter memory to hold more than ten glucose tests?
YES	NO	Do you want a meter that can record your insulin dose and other information as well?
YES	NO	Do you want a meter that can download its memory to a computer?
YES	NO	If your health care team downloads your meter information at your visits, is the meter compatible with your team's system?
YES	NO	Will you be using the meter at high altitudes or extremes of temperature? If so, are you able to use the meter under such varying conditions?
YES	NO	Do you have trouble getting a blood sample from your fingers? If so, does this meter require a very small sample of blood?
YES	NO	Would you prefer to use a test site other than your fingers, such as your arms or legs, to get a blood sample?
YES	NO	If you pay for test strips, are they affordable? (This will be your largest expense; the difference in cost between meters is small compared to the ongoing cost of strips.)
YES	NO	If the meter requires batteries, are the batteries easy to replace and convenient to find? (Some meter companies will give you a new meter when the batteries are low.)
YES	NO	Do you want a plasma-calibrated meter?

answer the questions, then make sure the meter you decide on meets most or all of your "Required?" responses.

Literally pages upon pages could be devoted to all the meter systems available on the market today. In addition, you could spend days, even weeks, traveling from pharmacy to pharmacy to see demonstrations of all the different meters. In general, no one store will have every single meter available for you to evaluate.

Keeping all of this in mind, you might find it easiest to begin your search via the Internet or with a good, nonbiased reference guide. One of the best references is the buyer's guide published every year in the December issue of the American Diabetes Association's *Diabetes Forecast* magazine. It can also be found on the Association's Web site at www.diabetes.org/diabetesforecast. All of the information is voluntarily supplied by the various product manufacturers. The American Diabetes Association does not review, endorse, or compare products but rather presents buying information about each category of products from those manufacturers who choose to provide it.

When Should I Test?

A recent study published in the *British Journal of Medicine* showed that frequent blood glucose testing did a better job of lowering blood glucose levels than any medication, diet, or exercise plan available to treat diabetes. It showed that the more often a person tested their blood glucose levels in a day, the better their blood glucose control overall. And further research has shown that the better the glucose control overall, the lower the risk of long-term complications of diabetes.

So, the best time to test is...as often as possible! Most people find that, generally, the best times to check blood glucose levels are just prior to meals and before going to sleep for the night. You may also find it extremely helpful to test one to two hours after you eat to see the effect of food on your glucose levels. By using your meter to check your blood glucose at different times of the day, you begin collecting valuable information and getting a good idea of how well your treatment program is working.

What Should My Numbers Be?

Your personal blood glucose goals will depend on your age, your type of diabetes and how long you've had it, any other health conditions you have, your lifestyle, and your desired level of control. You should check with your health care team to determine the best range of blood glucose levels for you. As a benchmark, the American Diabetes Association (ADA) has set a before-meal goal of 80–120 mg/dl and a bedtime goal of 100–140 mg/dl, as the standard of care for people with diabetes. The ADA recommends that if your before-meal levels are consistently lower than 80 or higher than 140 or your bedtime levels are consistently lower than 100 or higher than 160, you need a change in your treatment plan and should consult your diabetes team.

Also remember, when setting your blood glucose goals with your team, to take into account the type of meter you are using—whether it's a plasma-calibrated or whole-blood meter. The standards from the ADA are for whole-blood meters. If you are using a plasma-calibrated meter, you and your team need to add 12 percent to the stated goals. Always be sure to inform your health care team every time you change meters to determine if any changes are needed in your treatment program or in your target blood glucose ranges. In addition, if you change meter types or begin using more than one meter to do your testing, be sure you know how each meter is calibrated.

Finally, a word of caution: If your doctor does not ask you to do glucose testing or discourages the frequency of your testing, beware. You are not receiving the standard of care as recommended by the ADA and the American Association of Diabetes Educators.

Am I Doing This Right?

Obtaining a drop of blood is sometimes the most difficult part of blood glucose testing. Many meter

What Should I Be Trying to Achieve?

Remember: Set all goals together with your health care team!

LEVEL OF CONTROL	EXCELLENT		GOOD		POOR	
	whole blood	plasma	whole blood	plasma	whole blood	plasma
Before eating	60 to 100	70 to 110	100 to 140	110 to 155	over 180	over 200
After eating	100 to 140	110 to 155	140 to 180	155 to 200	over 220	over 245

manufacturers now provide lancing devices that can be adjusted to varying depths, depending on individual need, which helps reduce the pain of testing and improves the chances of obtaining an adequate sample.

Immediately before each test, make sure your hands are clean and free from anything that could influence your reading. When you wash your hands, use warm water. After drying, shake your hands below your waist and then squeeze, or milk, your test finger a few times before you lance a site. Make sure you use a new lancet before each test to ensure that it is clean and sharp. Place the lancet lightly against your finger, on the side of the pad (there are fewer nerve endings there), then push the lancet in to obtain your blood sample.

If you have ongoing problems obtaining an adequate sample to perform the test, talk with your health care team for suggestions. You may also want to explore using one of the alternate-site meters that allow you to obtain a blood sample from your arms or legs.

As previously discussed, testing is a vital part of your diabetes self-management. However, appropriate decisions regarding changes in your medications, eating, and level of activity can be made only if the results of your blood tests are accurate. According to an FDA-sponsored study, the main factors behind inaccurate readings appear to be inadequate training in the use of meters and a misunderstanding of the manufacturers' instructions leading to errors in the operation of the meters.

The most common errors that were found among meter-users were

- a failure to follow the manufacturer's procedures
- inadequate amount and placement of blood on the test strip
- failure to calibrate the meter
- lack of appropriate cleaning of the device
- the use of outdated test strips

Based on the FDA study, suggestions were made for reducing these errors. It was recommended that you

- obtain professional training and guidance for the use of your particular meter
- make sure you are using fresh strips and supplies
- clean your meter frequently (or use a meter that does not require cleaning)
- check your testing technique routinely with a professional
- follow the manufacturer's meter instructions carefully

If you faithfully follow these suggestions but suspect that your meter values are incorrect, reread the manufacturer's instructions. Then check the calibration of the meter and run a control test using the solution provided by the meter company. Repeat your blood glucose test again. If the meter's results still don't seem right, call your diabetes health professional or the meter manufacturer's 800 number, which is usually located on the back of the meter.

What if your meter reading doesn't match the laboratory's results for the same blood sample? Your meter reading is considered accurate if its results fall within 20 percent, plus or minus, of the laboratory results after any necessary conversions are made.

Remember that blood glucose meters and laboratory equipment measure glucose in different ways. Lab equipment uses only the plasma portion of blood to measure blood glucose, which means that the red blood cells are removed before glucose is measured. All blood glucose meters, on the other hand, measure the glucose level in whole blood, which is 12 percent lower. If you use a plasma-calibrated meter, you don't have to be concerned about that 12 percent difference, because your meter automatically makes that adjustment. Your results can be compared directly with those from the lab. And if they fall within 20 percent of each other, your testing is on target.

> ### Remember!
>
> Obtaining a drop of blood may be the most difficult part of blood glucose testing, but the reward is better diabetes control.

If, however, you use a noncalibrated whole-blood meter, you will need to do a mathematical conversion on the lab results in order to compare them to your own results. To do this, simply divide the lab results by 1.12. If your meter results fall within plus or minus 20 percent of the converted number, your testing is on target.

If, despite rechecking your calculations, the lab results and your meter results aren't close enough, report this to your diabetes care team.

What Do I Do With the Numbers?

If you are taking the time and going to the expense and trouble of testing your blood glucose levels, then you surely want something to come from your efforts. Try as you might, you will never be able to say for certain that you have complete control of your blood glucose levels. You will not be able to wake up one morning and confidently state that "All of my glucose levels will be under 140 today." You can, however, use the numbers that you get to help you confidently manage your diabetes.

To get the most out of your testing, you need a few pieces of information. First, make sure you know the correct way to perform a test. Next, know your target glucose levels, and figure out the best times to test your levels to give yourself and your team the most information. Finally, record your tests, even if your meter has a memory and you or your team can download your meter to retrieve the numbers.

Meter versus Lab

This example shows the calculation to figure the acceptable range when comparing your meter result to a lab result of 231.

Plasma-Calibrated Meter	Whole-Blood Meter	
$231 \times .20 = 46$ Variance	$231 \div 1.12 = 206$	Converted Result
$231 + 46 = 277$ Acceptable High	$206 \times .20 = 41$	Variance
$231 - 46 = 185$ Acceptable Low	$206 + 41 = 247$	Acceptable High
Acceptable Meter Range = 185 – 277	$206 - 41 = 165$	Acceptable Low
Which is ± 20% of 231	Acceptable Meter Range = 165 – 247	
	Which is ± 20% of 206	

When you keep a written record, not only do you have the time, date, and glucose levels that the meter records, but you also are able to record essential, and sometimes critical, information. Record the type and dose of each diabetes medicine you take and the time you take it. Do not fill your record book out ahead of time; your dose may change at some point or you may forget to take a dose. You want the record to accurately reflect what is happening to you. Record changes in your routine that may be affecting your glucose levels. You will want to note any unusual events such as changes in mealtimes or the amount of food eaten, changes in activity, illness, or unusual stress. Also be sure to record any low blood glucose events that occur.

With such detail, you and your team can identify glucose patterns and determine what causes your blood glucose fluctuations. You have enough information to manage the

diabetes and develop a plan to get your blood glucose levels to your target goal.

Keeping this record is vital. You and your health care professionals can use this information to make safe adjustments to your diet, level of activity, insulin, or oral medications. A well-kept record can help you and your team see patterns in your level of control. Always have your professionals "think out loud" when they make changes in your treatment plan. Ask them what they saw in your record of glucose levels to prompt a change and how they think the change will affect your future values. Make sure you understand their thinking and their logic. With time and practice, you may be able to do the same type of management.

Meter Choices Today and Tomorrow

When it comes to the future of blood glucose monitoring, the real excitement and anticipation centers around noninvasive meters, which measure blood glucose levels without needing a skin puncture to get a blood sample. Fortunately, the pipeline is full of breakthrough technologies that will revolutionize the monitoring of blood glucose and, as a result, the care of diabetes. A couple of early innovators in this area are already breaking out of the gate.

On July 15, 1999, the FDA granted premarket approval to MiniMed Inc. for its Continuous Glucose Monitoring System, which automatically monitors the glucose level in the patient with diabetes. A sensor is implanted just under the skin on the patient's abdomen for up to three days, recording glucose levels every five to six minutes during that time. The record is then downloaded in the doctor's office. From the resultant printouts, the doctor can analyze the glucose fluctuations that occurred during the three days and make recommendations about improving the patient's pattern of eating, medication administration, and activity level to improve blood sugar control. At present, the sensor does not provide on-demand blood sugar readings; the results must be downloaded. And it is currently available only for use under a doctor's care to monitor the patient's glucose levels over a 48- to 72-hour period. But MiniMed is currently devel-

The Future of Glucose Monitoring

Current methods of blood glucose monitoring require a blood sample. But researchers are trying to find new methods for people with diabetes to measure their blood sugar, methods that would not require a skin puncture.

The following are some of the noninvasive ways to measure glucose levels that are being studied:

- Shining infrared light through a person's forearm or finger

- Drawing glucose from the blood up through the skin using a low-level electrical current

- Measuring glucose levels in saliva or tears

oping a system for patient use that will display glucose readings on a screen and will also have an alarm that signals when glucose levels are dipping too low.

Cygnus, Inc., the makers of a breakthrough monitor called the GlucoWatch Biographer, was granted FDA approval on March 22, 2001, to market the watch as a prescription device for adults with diabetes. The GlucoWatch enables users to check their glucose levels at about 20-minute intervals throughout the day—without doing anything other than wearing the watchlike device and without feeling anything other than a tingling sensation. The GlucoWatch Biographer uses a low-frequency electrical current (supplied by a AAA battery) to draw out and measure glucose levels through the skin.

The race is on, and while these are the first competitors out of the gates, there are more than a dozen companies that have products soon to hit the market. Such devices promise to be the biggest step forward in diabetes self-management in 30 years.

CHAPTER 6

Your Diabetes Batting Average

Since the late 1970s, doctors have had access to laboratory tests that help them evaluate your blood glucose control over weeks or months. The two commonly used today are the glycohemoglobin and fructosamine tests. They don't replace the testing you do at home. Rather, they add to the information you and your doctor can use to assess your control.

What Is Glycohemoglobin?

Inside your red blood cells is a protein called *hemoglobin* that is responsible for carrying oxygen from the lungs to all the tissues in your body. Glucose attaches to hemoglobin inside the red blood cell, forming *glycohemoglobin*. Once the glucose attaches to the hemoglobin, it stays there as long as the red blood cell lives, generally about two or three months. Red blood cells don't all turn over, or die, at once (otherwise, you'd be without oxygen until they could be replaced). Old ones are constantly dying, and new ones are constantly being made. You might say that, at any one time, your red blood cells are a mix of the very old, the middle-aged, and the quite young, with more of them being on the younger side of their lives.

Normally, in someone who does not have diabetes, about 4 to 6 percent of the hemoglobin in their blood is coated in glucose. In the person with diabetes, who has blood glucose levels that are higher than normal, more glucose attaches to the hemoglobin molecules because there's more glucose circulating in the blood. For the person with diabetes, generally anywhere from less than 6 percent to more than 20 percent of their hemoglobin molecules are coated in glucose. The glycohemoglobin blood test measures this percentage. And because some of the hemoglobin molecules are older and some newer, the test results provide a view of the glucose levels over the past two to three months.

Glycohemoglobin actually refers to a family of glucose-coated hemoglobin molecules. One of these, the *hemoglobin A1c*, is thought to be the most stable member for the long-term measurement of glucose. In addition, because of its stability, it is unaffected by an immediate meal, so there's no need for the patient to fast before giving blood for the test. So, commonly, a glycohemoglobin test measures hemoglobin A1c (also written *HbA1c*).

Unfortunately, unlike cholesterol testing or blood pressure levels, there is no one standard value, no one correct range for the HbA1c. Each laboratory that conducts glycohemoglobin testing has a different range for a normal value. This problem of multiple "normals" will only be solved when all test values are measured on the same scale. Until then, to correctly use the HbA1c test, or any other glycohemoglobin test, you need to know the normal range values for the laboratory you use.

What Does an HbA1c Number Mean?

In general, when evaluating an HbA1c test, each percent increase in the hemoglobin A1c reflects an increase in average blood glucose of 30 mg/dl. So if an HbA1c of 6 percent is equal to an average blood glucose level of 120 mg/dl, then 7 percent would be equal to 150 mg/dl, 8 percent would equal 180 mg/dl, and so on. The American Diabetes Association recommends that the hemoglobin A1c goal be less than 7 percent for people with

What Does My Number Mean?

Your hemoglobin A1c value (HbA1c) is equal to an average blood glucose over the last two to three months. The American Diabetes Association recommends that your HbA1c value be below 7 percent to minimize long-term complications of diabetes.

Another formula you can use to determine your exact blood glucose average is:

$(HbA1c \times 30) - 60 =$ Average Blood Glucose

HbA1c %	AVERAGE BLOOD GLUCOSE (mg/dl)
13.0%	330
12.0%	300
11.0%	270
10.0%	240
9.0%	210
8.0%	180
7.0%	150
6.0%	120
5.0%	90
4.0%	60

diabetes. Most studies, however, have shown that only when the hemoglobin A1c is less than 6 percent is there no increase in diabetic complications.

Why Bother with Home Blood Tests?

As mentioned before, HbA1c testing is not a substitute for your own daily blood glucose monitoring. The HbA1c measures only the *average* glucose level over the past two to three months. Think of it as a baseball batting average: A batting average gives information about a player's overall success at bat. But you have no idea what kind of player he is from one day to the next. He could be hot one day and cold the next, or he could be a steady, dependable hitter. The same can be said for the HbA1c. The average of a glucose reading of 80 mg/dl and one of 120 mg/dl is 100 mg/dl and would reflect excellent control of diabetes. But the average of a glucose reading of 40 mg/dl and one of 160 mg/dl would also be 100 mg/dl and would not be good because a blood glucose reading of 40 mg/dl indicates hypoglycemia (a blood sugar level that is dangerously low).

Also remember that the blood glucose monitoring you do at home gives you specific information about your glucose level at the time of the test. It allows you to take immediate action to keep your blood glucose from going way too high or way too low. Based on the reading, you may decide that you need a snack, need more insulin, or need to check your urine for ketones. It's the overall effectiveness of these day-to-day decisions, based on your daily monitoring, that is reflected in your HbA1c.

There are some instances in which HbA1c testing can give you a false impression. Under certain conditions, for example, your hemoglobin molecules can have a shorter life span, resulting in artificially low HbA1c values. Such conditions include anemia caused by blood loss, pregnancy, kidney disease, and vitamin deficiencies. Rarely, the HbA1c value can be artificially high as a result of abnormalities in the hemoglobin; in such cases, HbA1c values can even reach levels above 50 percent.

If your HbA1c value does not seem to agree with the average of the values recorded by your blood-glucose meter (some meters provide you with an average of your readings over a specified period of time; otherwise, you can simply add up all the readings as you've recorded them in your log and divide that by the total number of entries to get your average), you should ask yourself the following questions:

- Am I testing frequently enough? Checking four times a day and occasionally one hour after meals should indicate your average value.
- Have I been testing long enough? You need to take the average of at least six-weeks' worth of blood-glucose readings to get a valid comparison to the HbA1c.
- Is my meter accurate? Use a single blood sample to compare the readings from your

meter against readings from your doctor's meter or from the lab (see Chapter 5 for more on this).

- Do I have a condition that may be shortening the life span of my hemoglobin molecules, such as anemia, kidney disease, or pregnancy?

If you've been testing long enough, if your meter's readings appear accurate, and if conditions that affect your hemoglobin have been ruled out, ask your doctor to redo the HbA1c. If there's still a discrepancy, you'll need to work with your diabetes care team to determine and correct the problem.

What About Fructosamine?

Fructosamine is made by the body in approximately the same manner as glycohemoglobin, only it involves the union of glucose with proteins (albumin and globulins) in your bloodstream. And like glycohemoglobin, it can be used to evaluate your level of blood glucose control. Because the turnover rate of these proteins is much faster than that of hemoglobin, the measurement of fructosamine provides a shorter term, more rapidly responding assessment of your glucose control. The fructosamine measurement reflects your average blood glucose level over the past two to

What Does My Number Mean?

Your fructosamine value is equal to an average blood glucose over the last two to three weeks. The American Diabetes Association has not set recommendations for fructosamine levels.

Another formula you can use to determine your exact blood glucose average is:

(Fructosamine x .8) − 80 = Average Blood Glucose

FRUCTOSAMINE	AVERAGE BLOOD GLUCOSE (mg/dl)
512	330
475	300
450	280
437	270
362	210
325	180
287	150
212	90
175	60
160	48

three weeks as opposed to the HbA1c value, which reflects your glucose control over the past two to three months.

Fructosamine levels are directly equal to the protein levels in your blood. Since the fructosamine level is not given as a percentage of total serum protein, a low level may indicate good control or it may simply indicate that the total level of protein in the blood is low.

Not all proteins are covered with glucose at the same rate. Normally, the protein present in your blood is largely albumin. However, in patients who have abnormally elevated levels of proteins other than albumin, the amount of glucose attaching to proteins may shift, affecting your fructosamine levels as well. In addition, alcohol and high levels of ascorbic acid (vitamin C) can interfere with the fructosamine test, so you should not drink alcohol nor take any vitamin C supplements for at least 24 hours prior to having your blood drawn for a fructosamine test. Finally, various diseases and stress states can change how fast protein is made and then how completely it is removed from the system, thus adversely affecting fructosamine results.

Fructosamine is usually measured in the laboratory, although a new combined glucosamine/fructosamine meter for home use has recently become available. Fructosamine testing may be done to assess diabetes control if an HbA1c test cannot be used because of other health conditions. And, since this test can reflect your control in the past two to three weeks, it can be particularly useful in assessing the effects of any recent adjustments made in your diabetes treatment.

CHAPTER 7

Food and Diabetes

Eating is essential to life, of course, but we eat for many reasons: out of hunger or habit, for pleasure, even as a way of dealing with emotions. A diagnosis of diabetes can make the simple act of eating seem overwhelmingly complicated. With education and experimentation, however, you can turn eating into a powerful tool for controlling diabetes.

There Is No Diabetic Diet Anymore

When you learned you had diabetes, you may have assumed you'd have to go on some special, restrictive diet. Perhaps you've heard about people with diabetes who had to give up all the foods they enjoyed or who stopped going to certain events or restaurants because there was nothing there they could eat. Well, cheer up. You don't need to follow a "diabetic diet" anymore.

A *diet* implies that you need to eat sparingly or according to prescribed rules. Diets also have a nasty habit of prohibiting rich, high-calorie, mouthwatering foods. Research shows that dieters often report overwhelming desires for the foods they're *not* supposed to eat on a diet and that they often give in to those cravings. Once they give in, they frequently overindulge. The traditional "diabetic diet" is really no different; indeed, it prescribes even greater food restrictions and pretty much dictates what foods are and are not allowed. Studies have shown, however, that those following a diabetic diet are no different than other dieters—they, too, eventually give in to their hungers and "binge" on "forbidden foods."

This diet/binge cycle is very common in those who diet frequently as well as in people with diabetes. It leads not only to failed weight-loss attempts but also to weight regain, yo-yo dieting, poor diabetes control, feelings of guilt, and constant food cravings.

The actual problem with diets—and the source of the ongoing diet/binge cycle and constant food cravings—is that dieting is based on four flawed assumptions:

1. The first flawed assumption is that eating is **always done in a continuous state of awareness.** For some people, however, eating comes close to being on the same level of consciousness as breathing. Have you ever found that you've polished off a whole box of crackers or some other snack and don't even remember taking the first bite? Somehow eating, like breathing, just happened without any thought. That's not to say that for periods of time a person can't focus intently on a diet, following every rule and detail. It's just that, in time, the spell will be broken and the person will drift back to old eating habits.

2. A diet presumes that we eat only to provide our bodies with fuel. But many people have strong expectations to have certain foods at certain times and places. Diets rarely take into consideration birthday or holiday celebrations, complete with traditional foods and cultural associations. Nor do they take into account Dad's classic Sunday morning brunch extravaganza or Grandma's candy drawer full of special treats. Only certain foods and food combinations will do at these times, otherwise it just doesn't seem the same.

3. Diets work on the belief that all of your emotional needs are met. Cravings for food and the need to eat can be the response to stresses in your life that need to be addressed. A diet discounts the need for comfort foods that calm and that are eaten in an attempt to soothe away life's troubles and turmoil. These foods have pleasurable tastes and textures and are used as rewards or to provide solace—a practice commonly begun in childhood and continued throughout life.

4. Diets operate on the idea that supply does not equal demand. In other words, as the supply of certain foods or food groups is limited by a prescribed diet, your desire or demand for these foods should not increase. However, just the opposite tends to be true. The deprivation of dieting sets you up to long for, think about, and plan your days around foods that you *can't, won't,* or *shouldn't* eat. It becomes a case of simply wanting what you can't have.

It's foolish and, in the end, self-defeating to deny the associations we have with food and the emotions certain foods evoke. Attempting to ignore these influences, which occurs anytime a diet is prescribed, sets people up for aberrant eating behaviors, such as food cravings, that result in binges and overeating. By trying to totally avoid certain foods, people instead tend to overconsume them in the end. For you, the person with diabetes, this can lead to additional problems.

You may skip your blood glucose testing or not record results—you may even go so far as to cancel medical appointments—because you figure you've "blown" your diet and testing would just be a reminder of your failure.

Rather than a restrictive diet, what you need are knowledge and information. You need to understand how food fuels and affects your body,

Out of Touch

A diet presumes that we eat only to fuel our bodies and tends to ignore the other factors that affect our eating habits.

especially your blood glucose levels, and then use that information, along with glucose monitoring, to choose a variety of foods—including the ones you enjoy most. To begin, then, you need to understand the fuels your body uses and how they affect your diabetes.

Fueling Your Body

Your body needs adequate amounts of six essential nutrients to function normally. Three of these nutrients—water, vitamins, and minerals—provide no energy and do not affect your blood glucose levels. The other three—carbohydrates, proteins, and fats—provide your body with the energy it needs to work. This energy is measured in calories. *Any* food that contains calories will cause your blood glucose levels to rise. And in order for your body to properly use these energy calories, it needs insulin.

NAME	TYPE
Glucose (Dextrose)	Simple Monosaccharide
Fructose	Simple Monosaccharide
Galactose	Simple Monosaccharide
Maltose (Malt Sugar)	Simple Disaccharide
Sucrose (Table Sugar)	Simple Disaccharide
Lactose (Milk Sugar)	Simple Disaccharide
Starch	Complex Polysaccharide
Fiber	Complex Polysaccharide

Whenever you eat, your food is digested and broken down to provide your body's primary fuel source, glucose. While all energy nutrients can be broken down into glucose, carbohydrates have a more direct and significant effect on blood glucose levels. Protein and fat have a slower, more indirect effect on those levels. Understanding this can help you predict how food will affect your blood glucose levels.

CARBOHYDRATES Commonly known as sugars and starches, carbohydrates are your body's main, and preferred, source of energy. They enter your bloodstream rapidly, are fairly predictable in the way they affect glucose, and are generally completely broken down in about two hours. There are three types of carbohydrates, simple carbohydrates (such as table sugar, honey, and fructose),

Types of Carbohydrates

WHAT IT LOOKS LIKE	WHERE IT IS FOUND
Single glucose unit	Fruits, some vegetables, honey, corn syrup
Single fructose unit	Table sugar, fruit, molasses, honey
Single galactose unit	Milk and dairy products
Two glucose units	Produced during the breakdown of starch
One glucose and one fructose unit hooked together	Table sugar, fruit, vegetables, grains
One glucose and one galactose unit hooked together	Milk and dairy products
Long chains of glucose units hooked together	Grains, legumes, potatoes
Long chains of glucose molecules hooked together that cannot be broken down by enzymes in your body	Fruits, vegetables, legumes

complex carbohydrates (such as bread, pasta, and potatoes), and fiber.

Nearly 100 percent of the simple and complex carbohydrates you eat break down into glucose; they do so at about the same speed, regardless of their source. There are two types of simple carbohydrates, *monosaccharides* (*mono* means one) and *disaccharides* (*di* means two). Monosaccharides, such as glucose and fructose, are single sugar units. Disaccharides consist of two sugar units; sucrose, or table sugar, is a combination of a glucose and a fructose.

Complex carbohydrates are referred to as *poly-saccharides* (*poly* means many) because they consist of many long chains of glucose units hooked together. Complex carbohydrates are found in grains, fruits, beans, and vegetables. When complex carbohydrates are digested by your body, they are broken down into glucose, the simplest form of energy used by your body and your brain. The sugar in an apple and the sugar in your sugar bowl, therefore, are really the same as far as your body is concerned. The body breaks down and utilizes the glucose from each item in identical ways, and it has no way of knowing whether the energy came from a simple carbo-hydrate or a complex carbohydrate.

However, people with diabetes often think, or have been taught, they cannot or should not have any simple carbohydrates, or sugar, in their diet. Sugar has traditionally been viewed as a forbid-den food and a real danger for people with dia-betes. After all, the blood "sugar" is high, so why complicate matters? Doctors and dietitians always assumed that since sugar was a simple carbohydrate, it must be more quickly digested and absorbed into the blood than complex carbo-hydrates such as the starch in potatoes and breads. They further assumed that simple sugars would most likely cause a larger rise in blood glucose levels.

Well, doctors, dietitians, and all the food police were wrong! Multiple studies have shown that all foods increase blood sugar and that simple carbohydrates don't increase your glucose levels any higher or faster than other carbohydrates. In 1994, these conclusive studies led the American Diabetes Association to change its nutritional recommendations. The recommendations now say, "Scientific evidence has shown that the use of sucrose as part of the meal plan does not impair blood glucose control in individuals with Type 1 or Type 2 diabetes." It is now generally recognized that the total carbohydrate in your diet, not the source of the carbohydrate, is what significantly influences your blood glucose levels.

How Sweet!

Sugar used to be a forbidden food for people with diabetes, but research has shown that it doesn't deserve that bad rap.

Fiber is made up mostly of complex carbohydrates—so complex, in fact, that they cannot be broken down by enzymes in your body. There are two types of fiber, soluble and insoluble. Soluble fiber dissolves in water, while insoluble fiber does not. Soluble fiber, found in oats, barley, cereals, apples, and citrus fruits, delays glucose absorption, lowers cholesterol, and decreases the speed at which food moves through your intestines. Insoluble fiber, found in all fruits, vegetables, legumes, and seeds, also delays glucose absorption and slows the breakdown of starch, but it increases the speed at which food moves through your intestines.

PROTEIN The second major nutrient needed by your body is protein. The protein in the foods you eat (meats, poultry, fish, beans, dairy products, and eggs) is broken down into amino acids by your body; only about 50 percent of it is eventually changed into glucose. This is a long process, and it takes about three to five hours after a meal for the protein you have eaten to have any impact on your blood glucose. When carbohydrates and fats are not available or are in short supply (as when you don't eat between your evening meal and breakfast the next morning), amino acids can be made into glucose as a backup source of energy.

FAT The third nutrient needed by your body is fat. Yes, fat is important and your body needs it. Fat is used to maintain healthy skin and hair, to carry fat-soluble vitamins through your body, and to serve as a major source of energy when you take in fewer calories than your body needs. Fats are changed by your body into fatty acids, which are an important source of energy for your muscles and heart. It generally takes about six to eight hours for the fat in food to be digested, and its components are released very slowly into your blood. In the end, only about five to ten percent of the fat you eat is changed into glucose, so it has little direct impact on your blood glucose levels. Indirectly, however, fat does play a role in elevating blood glucose. Fat blocks the action of insulin (its fatty acids increase your insulin resistance) and increases the time it takes for food to travel through your intestines. This means that your dinner of fried chicken, mashed potatoes, gravy, and biscuits may not significantly affect your glucose reading before you go to bed. During the night, however, when the fat-laden, slow-moving food finally hits your system and the fat doesn't let your insulin work very well, your blood glucose level rises. In the morning, you are greeted by a whopper of a blood glucose number.

Alcohol: Carbohydrate, Protein, or Fat?

Actually, none of the above. Alcohol is viewed more as a toxic product by your body than as an energy source. It is a poisonous product that needs to be broken down, detoxified, and removed from your blood as quickly as possible to prevent it from accumulating and destroying the body's cells and organs.

When you drink, alcohol passes very quickly from your stomach and intestines into your blood without being broken down. Enzymes in your liver then do the job of breaking down the alcohol, but this process takes time. Your liver can metabolize alcohol only at a set rate, regardless of how much you have had to drink. If you drink alcohol faster than your liver can break it down, the excess alcohol moves through your bloodstream to other parts of your body until it can be metabolized. Your brain cells are affected by this excess, impairing brain function and causing alcohol intoxication.

Whether or not you have eaten and the type of food you have eaten are two factors that influence how quickly alcohol is absorbed into your bloodstream. Since alcohol can be processed only at a certain rate by your liver, slowing down the absorption (how quickly alcohol appears in your blood) can be beneficial. How fast your stomach empties into your intestines is the primary control for how quickly alcohol is absorbed. The higher the fat content of a meal, the slower the emptying and the longer the absorption process. A study even found that people who drank alcohol after a meal that included fat, protein, and carbohydrates absorbed the alcohol about three times more slowly than when they drank the same amount of alcohol on an empty stomach.

Aside from the intoxication alcohol can cause, the process of breaking down alcohol cuts ahead of other processes that are on the liver's

Toxic Toast

The body sees alcohol as a poison that must be broken down, detoxified, and removed from your blood as soon as possible.

agenda. Normally, if your blood glucose level starts to drop, your liver responds by changing stored energy, glycogen, into glucose. This glucose then helps you avoid or slow down a low blood glucose reaction. However, since your body sees alcohol as a poison, it wants to clear it from your blood as quickly as possible. In fact, it is so busy processing the alcohol that it will not make or release any glucose until the alcohol is gone from your system.

The intoxication and the inability to produce glucose can put you at risk for a number of different problems, including a severe hypoglycemic (low blood glucose) reaction (see Chapter 10). This can be compounded even further if you have

consumed enough alcohol to impair your judgment; this impairment can stunt or even erase
your ability to notice symptoms of hypoglycemia.
In addition, because the symptoms of
hypoglycemia mimic intoxication, a low blood
glucose reaction can easily be confused with
drunkenness, delaying treatment even further.

So, do you have to abstain from alcohol in order
to control blood glucose? Can you have a beer
with your pizza or a glass of wine with your
spaghetti? There is no one right answer. You need
to discuss it with your diabetes care team. Your
history regarding alcohol consumption needs to
be reviewed, the medications that you take need
to be assessed for potentially harmful interactions
with alcohol, and your diabetes control needs to
be evaluated. Should you receive the green light
from your providers, keep the following in mind:

1 Drink only if your diabetes is under good
control.

Alcohol can make some diabetes problems worse.
Alcohol can accumulate in nerve cells, intensify-
ing the damage done to them by the high glucose
levels and, therefore, worsening neuropathy. It
also raises triglycerides, blood pressure, and the
risk of cataracts. If you have frequent hypogly-

cemia or a past history of severe hypoglycemia, alcohol may be too big a risk for you.

2. Drink in moderation.

The breakdown of alcohol by your liver is a slow process, so the amount of alcohol you drink needs to be controlled to prevent accumulation and subsequent intoxication. Moderation generally means no more than one to two drinks once or twice a week. A single drink is defined as 12 ounces of beer, 4 ounces of wine, or $1^{1}/_{2}$ ounces of distilled liquor. Remember, alcohol has no nutrients, only energy (calories), most of which your body stores as fat.

3. Do not skip a meal or eat less when drinking.

Have your drink either with a meal or shortly after eating. Never drink on an empty stomach, and do not skip meals or substitute alcohol for your usual meal or snack.

4. Always carry some form of identification.

It is preferred that your identification indicate that you have diabetes. This lets people know that your erratic behavior or loss of consciousness may not be due to intoxication but rather to severe hypoglycemia.

5. Never drink alone.

Inform those around you that you have diabetes, and teach them the signs and symptoms of hypo-glycemia. This way, at least they may think of the possibility of hypoglycemia and not ignore or delay treatment of a hypoglycemic reaction.

6. Remain sober.

Since alcohol has a relaxing effect, it can impair your judgment. You need to eat your meals and take your medication on time and test your blood sugar on a regular basis.

7. Test your blood glucose frequently.

Understand how alcohol affects you by testing prior to drinking, after drinking, and the next day. Be sure to always test your blood glucose before going to sleep. And never give yourself extra insulin or take extra diabetes pills to treat a high blood glucose reading and then go to bed. You could become dangerously hypoglycemic as you sleep and never even notice it.

What About Sweeteners?

There are two types of sweeteners on the market today: those that have calories, called nutritive sweeteners, and those that have no calories, called artificial, or nonnutritive, sweeteners. Only the nutritive sweeteners affect your blood glucose directly, but you'll still need to pay attention to the other ingredients in foods that use artificial sweeteners.

NUTRITIVE SWEETENERS The simple carbohydrates sucrose and fructose are the most common nutritive sweeteners used; both contribute calories and influence your blood glucose levels.

Sugar alcohols, also called polyols, contain calories and carbohydrates and are often used as substitute sweeteners, especially in candy. While the name implies two seemingly forbidden words, sugar and alcohol, sugar alcohols are neither sugars nor alcoholic substances in the common sense of the term. (The scientific definition of alcohol is simply "a processed liquid.") Sugar alcohols are the commercially produced, processed liquids from sucrose, glucose, and starches (polysaccharides). They also occur naturally in plants such as fruits and berries. Common sugar alcohols include sorbitol, mannitol, maltitol, and xylitol.

Another sugar alcohol, called *hydrogenated starch hydrolysate*, is made by partially breaking down corn, wheat, or potato starch and then adding hydrogens, at a high temperature and

Nutritive Sweeteners

Sucrose (white sugar)	It is very versatile in terms of use, readily available, and inexpensive.
Glucose	It has limited use because of a lower level of sweetness and is mainly used in candies to provide smoothness at high temperatures.
Fructose	It is sweeter than sucrose in cold liquids, but in warm liquids and solid foods, it is only as sweet as sucrose. It enhances fruit flavors.
Honey	It is nutritionally similar to sucrose and is chemically formed from nectar by bees. It has a very distinctive flavor and a very high water content.
Lactose	It is the sugar found in milk and is a disaccharide, made up of glucose and galactose linked together. It has a very low sweetness, which limits its uses alone, but it is often used in combination with intense sweeteners as a "filler." Lactose intolerance is common and occurs in people who lack the digestive enzyme lactase, which breaks apart the glucose and galactose units.
Sorbitol Mannitol	They are sugar alcohols and are about half as sweet as sucrose, which limits their uses. They are incompletely absorbed by your body, so they add fewer calories and carbohydrates to the food being eaten. Because of incomplete digestion, they can cause diarrhea, gas, and bloating when used in large quantities. They are more expensive than sucrose.
Xylitol Maltitol	They are sugar alcohols. Both are about as sweet as sucrose and so are more widely used, especially in candies and baked goods. They are incompletely absorbed, so they have fewer calories and carbohydrates. They also may cause diarrhea, gas, and bloating when used in large quantities.
Hydrogenated Starch Hydrolysate	It's the "complex carbohydrate" of sugar alcohols. It's made up of large chains of polysaccharides plus hydrogen put together under heat and pressure to form very stable, complex sugar alcohols. Widely used in candies and with low-calorie, nonnutritive sweeteners.

under pressure, to the partially broken-down mixture. As a result, they contain higher quantities of hydrogenated polysaccharides as well as sorbitol, mannitol, maltitol, and xylitol. They are kind of the "complex carbohydrate" of the sugar alcohols. They are used in a variety of products, especially sugar-free candies, because they do not crystallize. They also blend well with flavors and can be used with low-calorie sweeteners.

As a group, sugar alcohols are not completely absorbed and used by your body as energy, so they contribute fewer calories and carbohydrates compared to the same amount of other nutritive sweeteners, such as sucrose. For this reason, they are referred to as reduced-energy or low-energy sweeteners. However, because they are not completely absorbed, they can produce unpleasant side effects such as diarrhea, bloating, and gas when consumed in excess.

ARTIFICIAL SWEETENERS Artificial sweeteners are man-made, intensely sweet products that are most commonly used in reduced-calorie foods and beverages. They are termed nonnutritive sweeteners because they add very few, if any, calories and carbohydrates to the foods they sweeten. Because such a small amount of these sweeteners is needed to produce a "sweet" taste

Nonnutritive Sweeteners

Saccharin (Sweet'N Low)	It provides no energy. It is 200 to 700 times sweeter than sucrose but has a bitter, metallic aftertaste.
Aspartame (Nutrasweet)	It is made up of two amino acids linked together. The amino acids break apart when they are heated, and the sweetness deteriorates, so it can only be used in cold foods and drinks. It is 160 to 220 times sweeter than sucrose. It cannot be used by persons with phenylketonuria.
Acesulfame K (Sweet One)	It is an organic salt consisting of carbon, nitrogen, oxygen, hydrogen, sulphur, and potassium atoms. It is 200 times sweeter than sucrose and is heat stable.
Sucralose (Splenda)	It is the only nonnutritive sweetener made from sugar. Through a special method, three hydrogen-oxygen groups on the sugar molecule are replaced with three chlorines. It is used as a sugar replacement and as an additive in a variety of desserts, confections, and nonalcoholic beverages. It is 600 times sweeter than sucrose, and its sweetening power is not reduced by heating.

in foods, they are also referred to as high-intensity sweeteners. The major artificial sweeteners are Nutrasweet (aspartame), Sweet One (acesulfame K), Splenda (Sucralose), and Sweet'N Low (saccharin).

IS IT REALLY "SUGAR FREE"? How is it that a manufacturer can slap a big "Sugar Free" label on the front of a box of cookies even though the product contains sugar? The answers: "Quite simply" and "quite legally." All that the term "sugar free" means is that a product contains less than .5 gram of sugar in a serving—and "sugar" in this context is defined as sucrose. That's right. "Sugar free" simply means that table sugar or cane sugar is not in the item. The manufacturer can add fructose and any other nutritive sweetener and still call it "sugar free."

As a result, it is not unusual for a "sugar free" product to actually contain more total carbohydrates than the "regular" version of the same product. For the person with diabetes, that means that the "sugar free" item will actually raise blood glucose levels *more* than the regular version of the food would. The same is also true for

Sweet Truth

Keep in mind that the "sugar free" version of a food may actually contain more total carbohydrates than the regular version.

many "fat free" foods. They truly have less than .5 gram of fat per serving, but when the fat is removed or not used in processing, simple carbohydrates may be added instead. So some "fat free" and "fat free, sugar free" products actually have more carbohydrates and therefore will raise blood glucose levels higher than the regular item would.

Also understand that a "sugar free" food is not necessarily one that is calorie free, low in calories, or low in simple carbohydrates. Some foods may even have sugar listed on the label, even though the label also says "sugar free." Milk is a good example. On the food label for milk, you will find that one serving contains 13 grams of sugar. Milk doesn't contain sucrose, or table sugar. It does, however, contain the naturally occurring simple carbohydrate (sugar) called lactose. The point is that because a product is labeled "sugar free" doesn't mean you can ignore its potential effect on your blood glucose levels.

That's why it's important to look more closely at food labels to check the actual calorie and carbohydrate counts. As you look at any product, the middle part of the food label contains information on carbohydrates, fat, protein, and other nutrients. This section has the greatest amount of information for the person with diabetes who is trying to figure out the connection between food and blood glucose levels.

On all labels, carbohydrates are measured in grams. As you've learned, gram for gram, all carbohydrates have the same effect on blood sugar levels. So use the food labels to compare foods in terms of their total carbohydrate. Make sure the serving sizes you are comparing are similar. Then choose the product that best fits into your carbohydrate goals (which you'll learn about shortly). In addition, monitoring your blood sugar before and after eating or drinking will help you see a food's effect on your blood sugar.

The Food Choices Are Yours

Okay, so now you have an understanding of the nutrients in food that affect your blood glucose. To successfully use your knowledge of food as part of your diabetes self-care, you need to make personal food choices that are compatible with your blood glucose goals and your tastes. Since carbohydrates obviously have the greatest direct effect on glucose levels, determining the amount of carbohydrates that your body can manage well is a cornerstone in your glucose management. It's simple, really. But before you begin, you should take a close look at your habits and your perceptions and preconceptions about food and eating; they can make eating much more complicated than it need be. Adjusting them can allow you to enjoy the freedom that simplicity brings—and allow you to enjoy eating while you control your diabetes.

According to multiple studies, the amount of carbohydrate in what you are eating is more important than the type of carbohydrate (simple versus complex) in terms of blood glucose. In other words, a carbohydrate is a carbohydrate is a carbohydrate. So while a snack of one large,

Some of the Foods that Contain Carbohydrates

Rice	Pasta	Breads
Cereals	Fruits	Juices
Vegetables	Milk & Milk Products	Nuts
Candy	Cakes	Pies
Chips & Pretzels	Beans	Popcorn
Crackers	Sodas	Pancakes & Waffles
Tortillas	Cookies	Jams & Jellies

FOODS THAT DO NOT HAVE CARBOHYDRATES

Meats & Fats

extra-chunky chocolate chip cookie may seem "bad" and a snack consisting of three small sugar-free cookies may seem "good," your body can't tell the difference between the two if both snacks have the same amount of carbohydrates. Both will raise your glucose level the same amount.

You may be thinking to yourself "No way." Your preconceptions about food may be telling you that eating extra-chunky cookies or a candy bar *must* raise your glucose levels higher than eating a baked potato or sugar-free pudding. Perhaps your experience even backs you up on that. The culprit in this apparent discrepancy, though, is not the type of carbohydrate. Your preconceptions—and the total amount of carbohydrate you consume—are really to blame.

Consider this: Generally, when, what, and why you eat has as much (or more) to do with habit or craving as it has to do with hunger. So while you may eat just one baked potato, you may be driven to eat an entire candy bar, not because you are still hungry after finishing half of it, but because it just tastes so good and it has been so long since you've allowed yourself to have chocolate. As a matter of fact, it's been so long that you may feel entitled to have two candy bars. So you end up eating more candy—and more total carbohydrate. It's that larger amount of carbohydrate, not the source of the carbohydrate, that sends your glucose soaring.

The kind of deprivation that might have driven you to eat that second candy bar can drive your eating in other ways as well. There's nothing that can heighten your desire for a food quite like being told you cannot have it. So, you have a nice lunch, followed by a sugar-free cookie... followed by three extra-chunky chocolate chip cookies. You figure you've eaten what you're supposed to eat, now you're getting what you *really* want. You then blame your elevated glucose levels on the extra-chunky cookies. While they are a contributor, they are not the problem. If you had ended your lunch with the extra-chunky cookie you wanted in the first place, rather than the one you were "supposed to have," your glucose level would have been lower in the end. It was your drive to get what you want, and your initial self-imposed deprivation, that set you up to fail. And it's this kind of restrictive thinking that can make some foods seem off-limits or more dangerous in terms of glucose control.

Deprivation can also lead to desperation, and desperate times lead to desperate measures. For example, perhaps you're always the last one in your household to go to bed, staying up well past the others because you're "just not tired yet." Or perhaps you decline dinner invitations and evenings out because you are "too tired"; you send everyone else out, leaving you home, alone. Now, in quiet solitude, you can eat in peace, without anyone commenting or watching your intake. You're like the escaped convict, trying to outrun the law as fast and as far as you can before you are captured again by the food police and thrown back into deprivation jail.

Like preconceptions, your eating habits can also interfere with your dietary diabetes management. Food habits and eating patterns are developed over years and are often ingrained from child-hood. You do something one way because that is just how it is done. You finish the food on the plate because you shouldn't waste food. You eat all the food on the plate because you paid for it, someone else paid for it, or it is free. You eat because the label on your pill bottle tells you that you must eat in order to take them. You eat because it is time and the clock tells you so. These habits involving your eating have very little to do with hunger or your blood glucose levels but have become the rules by which your eating is driven.

To end this cycle of deprivation and to be able to truly use your food choices to help control your diabetes, you need to make all food equal and not make any food off-limits. You need to convince yourself once and for all that there are no good foods and bad foods. There are merely foods that affect your blood glucose in different ways. This will eliminate your feelings of deprivation. If you know you can have candy whenever you want, the drive to eat it because you are unsure if or when you'll ever get another opportunity will disappear. You'll be able to eat because you are hungry for a certain item, not because you'll never see it again.

Instead of eating because you want to or are supposed to, ask yourself instead if you are hun-

It's Not What You're Eating, It's How Much You're Eating

45 GRAMS OF CARBOHYDRATES	AMOUNT YOU WOULD NORMALLY EAT	AMOUNT OF CARBOHYDRATES ACTUALLY EATEN
2 baked potatoes	1 potato—It's the reasonable, standard amount.	23
1 regular-sized candy bar	2 candy bars—one because you crave it and one because you've blown your diet anyway, so you might as well go for it.	90
3 pieces of whole-wheat toast	2 pieces of toast—because the toaster holds two slices. In addition, you have to finish the second piece because "there are children starving somewhere."	30
1½ cups of a sugar-frosted cereal	3 cups—Who decided that ¾ cup of cereal was a serving size? In a country where we "super size" everything, small is sure to leave me hungry.	90

gry. You have an internal wisdom that lets you know when you need to eat and when you need to stop. While this system has many drivers, one is your blood glucose level. When your blood glucose is on the low side, you become hungry; at higher levels, hunger is absent. (If you find yourself having to eat when you're not hungry because you need to take your medication with food, discuss this fact with your health care team.) Eliminating the deprivation and examining your habits will let you find the carbohydrate balance that allows you to maintain your glucose goals. It will help you change your relationship with food for the better and improve your diabetes control.

Explore Your Food Options

To further understand your diabetes and your blood glucose variations, you must pay attention to how foods act in your body. You need to approach this just like a scientist, collecting data about blood glucose and types and amounts of foods, then drawing conclusions based on that data.

The first step is for you to eat normally, absolutely normally. Eat what you want, when you want it, and exactly how much you want. Figure out which foods contain carbohydrates and count the number of carbohydrates that you are eating throughout an entire day. Take detailed and honest notes.

Along with it, you need to test your blood glucose levels. Testing will allow you to see how well your insulin (either that you have injected or that your body has produced) matches the carbohydrates that you have eaten. In all cases, insulin works with the food you eat. It is this balance that is one of the key aspects of diabetes control. If you eat too much food for the insulin that is available, your glucose level will be too high; if you eat too little, your glucose level will be too low.

Test before you eat and then one, two, three, and four hours after the meal. As a general guideline, aim for a pre-meal glucose goal of 80-120 mg/dl. One hour after the meal, you want a glucose reading less than 180 mg/dl; two hours after the meal, less than 160 mg/dl; three hours after, less than 140; and at four hours, or prior to your next meal, back to 80-120 mg/dl. Just as you know the number of miles per gallon (mpg) of gas you can travel in your car, you will gradually begin to figure out your body's *cpm*, or *carbohydrates per meal*—the distance your body can travel each time you eat a certain amount of carbohydrates.

You may find that eating foods that contain only carbohydrates causes your blood glucose to rise rapidly or stay too high after the meal. Carbohydrates in combination with varying amounts of fat and/or protein will affect your blood glucose differently. In addition, you may discover that high-fat foods elevate your blood glucose levels as well.

It is important to know that any food has the ability to make blood sugar levels rise, but different types of food choices as well as amounts of foods will result in different levels of blood sugar in your body. You may find that overeating (eating when you are not hungry) makes blood sugar levels increase rapidly and stay too high. Overeat-

Keeping Track

It's important to track how your blood glucose level responds to different foods. And since carbohydrates (starches and sugars) have the biggest effect on blood sugar, it's especially important to determine their impact on your blood sugar levels. For example, see how your level increases after you eat similar amounts of potatoes, pasta, or corn. And do the same with similar foods: Compare sugar-sweetened cereals with those that contain relatively little sugar.

In a journal, record what you ate and its carbohydrate content, as well as your blood glucose levels just before you ate and at one hour, two hours, three hours, and four hours after eating. You're aiming for these numbers:

Pre-meal glucose level: 80–120

1 hour after a meal: <180

2 hours after a meal: <160

3 hours after a meal: <140

4 hours after a meal: 80–120

ing may not allow insulin to do its job properly. Listening to your body's internal hunger cues and respecting fullness causes the blood sugar to go up more slowly and not reach as high a level. This allows insulin to do its job properly and keep blood sugars at a healthy level. This type of balanced eating helps control diabetes and helps you feel better.

As you experiment and test your blood glucose, try a wide variety of foods. Enjoy different types of carbohydrates, from pasta to potatoes, biscuits to green beans, and bread to blueberries. Eat a variety of proteins, from eggs to cheese and ground turkey to prime rib. Try various types of fats, from butter to margarine and sour cream to mayonnaise. Look for patterns in the ways various foods and food combinations affect your glucose.

Eating a wide variety will also help ensure that you get the nutrients you need—not just the carbohydrate, protein, and fat but also the vitamins and minerals that are essential to overall good health. In addition, the multitudes of tastes, textures, and colors will continue to enhance your eating pleasure.

> ### Vary Well
>
> It's important to eat a wide variety of foods to get the vitamins and minerals as well as fat, protein, and carbohydrate your body needs.

If you need some advice on expanding your food horizons or if you have concerns related to losing excess body fat or controlling other health problems such as heart disease, sit down with your diabetes care team. They will be able to provide a wealth of suggestions that can help you. Remember, though, that even for these other conditions, "diets" are not the answer. Cutting out food groups or making certain foods off-limits will make these endeavors fail as well. Your educator or dietitian can provide suggestions for tuning into your hunger, decreasing overeating, balancing your diet, comparing various foods, and making relatively painless substitutions that can improve your health without making you feel deprived. Be sure to seek and take advantage of the practical guidance they can provide.

Eat With Joy, Pleasure, and Awareness

There truly is an alternative to diets, those externally imposed, dictatorial dietary restrictions that result in those overpowering cravings and abandonment of self-care. Work to understand the effect of foods on your blood glucose levels. Know that restricting foods creates "good" and "bad" food labels and that these terms imply guilt and assign emotional labels to food.

Come to learn how you use food for comfort and calming. When you find yourself eating and you recognize that you are not hungry, ask yourself why. What is it that you need right now? Do you need a break from that project? Would a walk, a bath, a call to a friend, or some quiet time make you feel better? Are you craving the food because you've been restricting yourself and trying to stay away from that food? Listen to your thoughts. Then listen to your body; it knows what it needs.

As Hippocrates stated, "Thy food shall be thy remedy." In regards to diabetes, nothing is closer to the truth. While food is a major aspect of diabetes management, it is also a part of many important and enjoyable aspects of our lives. With an understanding of how food affects and interacts with diabetes and our emotional self, you can use it in a positive way to affect your glucose control, your self-care, and your overall health.

CHAPTER 8

Activity

The difference between exercise and activity is that exercise is something you do three times a week and hate, while activity is something you do three times a week and like."

—Allen King, M.D.

Moving Toward Better Control

The three cornerstones of diabetes treatment are food, medications, and activity. Of these three, activity is often a first choice by the person with diabetes. An investment in a physically active life is generally inexpensive, convenient, and easy and usually reaps great rewards in terms of glucose control and a general feeling of well-being.

If you recall, whenever you actively use a muscle, you burn both fatty acids and glucose. During and after periods of activity, the falling glucose level is sensed by the beta cells in your pancreas, and they relax their output of insulin. This takes the strain of excessive insulin production off your beta cells. In addition, the lower insulin levels signal your liver to empty its glucose reserves (glycogen) into the blood to supply the muscles with needed energy. As the activity continues, the liver converts amino acids, lactic acid, and fats into glucose in order to supply glucose to the working muscles. If the activity continues long enough, even the body's fat cells get in on the game. They compensate for the reduced fatty acid levels in your blood by converting their triglycerides to fatty acids.

When all of these steps are considered, using your muscles is the perfect treatment for diabetes. You lower your blood glucose levels, you lower the fatty acid levels in your blood, and you reduce the workload on your pancreas. And, unless you are on a medication that can cause hypoglycemia, increased levels of activity will not cause your blood glucose level to fall below normal.

Before You Get Going

There are some risks to increasing your activity level. However, remaining sedentary is no bargain either. It does nothing to help your glucose control, your weight management, or your overall well-being. The best way to gain the benefits of increased physical activity and minimize potential risks is to understand and evaluate those risks up front and take steps to prevent problems before they occur.

HYPOGLYCEMIA For people with diabetes who take medication or insulin, hypoglycemia is a concern. Whenever you are physically active, glucose is pouring into muscle tissue, supplying it with needed energy. This glucose continues to pour into your muscles even when you have stopped the activity. In order to build and provide a reservoir of glucose in the muscles for future physical activity, your body takes in glucose from the blood and uses it to restock the muscles' stores of glycogen. As a result, a hypoglycemic reaction can occur not only during periods of activity but up to 24 hours later.

Some people with diabetes who have frequently experienced hypoglycemia begin to associate any form of activity with a loss of glucose control. For such individuals, a lack of glucose testing may keep them in the dark about how their body reacts to activity. As a result, they are unprepared for the low blood glucose level that occurs when

Reasons to Be More Active

- Lower my blood glucose
- Lower my blood pressure
- Maintain a stable weight
- Lower my blood fats
- Improve cardiovascular fitness
- Feel good

they mow the lawn, say, or when they take a brisk walk through the park. When such a low occurs, they may grab a handful of jelly beans to treat the low, only to find their glucose level skyrocketing as a result. So they take extra insulin or medication at dinner to treat the high, but the blood-glucose roller-coaster ride continues with another low before they go to bed. These fluctuations create great confusion and frustration, leaving these individuals upset and scared. Activity, they may decide, is not worth the cost of seemingly worse control. For such individuals, more frequent blood glucose testing can help them better understand their body's response to exercise and prepare for it by adjusting medication or food intake.

HEART DISEASE Another risk to assess is heart disease. As you've already learned, coronary heart disease is very common in people with diabetes, affecting perhaps as many as 50 percent of them. The risk factors for it include age, blood pressure, blood fats, the presence of protein in your urine, the length of time you have had diabetes, and your family history. So before you begin increasing your level of activity, it would be wise to consult your doctor and, if appropriate, have an exercise tolerance test. This test is performed as you exercise on a treadmill and reflects your heart's ability to work under stress. Your chances of a positive result from the treadmill test (which would indicate heart disease) increase with each risk factor you have. Even if you are at increased risk or have a positive test, you will likely still be able to increase your physical activity; you will just need to work more closely with your diabetes care team to set safe guidelines for activity and, perhaps, to determine if medications to lower your heart risk are in order.

DIABETES COMPLICATIONS Before you increase your activity level, you should also consider diabetic complications. Certain types of activity may not be wise choices for some people.

Any activity that includes straining, such as weight lifting, can dramatically increase your blood pressure during the activity, further aggra-

> ## Caution!
>
> Before increasing your level of physical activity, check with your doctor and, if necessary, get an exercise tolerance test.

vating hypertension. To minimize any potential problems, your blood pressure must be well controlled before increasing your activity level.

Proliferative retinopathy is also aggravated by straining, which increases the pressure in the weakened arteries of the eye. Activities such as weight lifting that involve straining and any activity that involves jarring or rapid head motions may also cause an acute hemorrhage in already weakened eye vessels. For this reason, it is important to have your eyes examined for retinopathy before starting an exercise program and then have them rechecked annually.

If you have significant nerve disease in your feet, you may not be able to feel injuries to your feet, the most common of which are blisters. This does not mean you cannot exercise, but it means that you need to have your feet checked by your doctor first and you must observe good daily foot care at home, including inspecting your feet for sore spots and minor injuries.

Guidelines for Activity

The following guidelines can help you increase your activity level safely. Be sure to work with your diabetes care team, too, so they can monitor you and provide specialized advice for your specific situation.

SCREENING First, be screened by your doctor for any possible problems before you start any type of activity. This exam should include a treadmill test for those people with diabetes who are more

than 35 years of age, an eye examination for proliferative retinopathy, a urine examination for
protein, and a medical evaluation of your feet.

TYPE OF ACTIVITY Once you've received your
team's okay for exercise, choose activities that fit
your condition, your lifestyle, and your tastes.
Running or jogging may be out of the question for
people with significant neuropathy, and a contact
sport or any activity that requires straining is not
a wise choice if you have uncontrolled blood
pressure or proliferative retinopathy. Many people with diabetes, especially those who have not
been physically active for a while, find that easy,
low-impact activities such as walking and swim-
ming are perfect.

Whatever you choose, make sure the activities are
enjoyable for you and take into account your
abilities and condition. The activities don't even
have to be "exercises" in the traditional sense, as
long as they get you moving. Square dancing,
walking your dog, riding your bike, gardening, and
even walking the golf course all count. Vary them
so that you don't get bored or fall prey to easy
excuses. Choose some that can be done with
others and some that can be done alone; some
that can be done indoors, some that can be done
outdoors; some that can be done when your

schedule is light, and some that you can fit in when you're strapped for time.

TIME, INTENSITY, AND DURATION Begin each exercise period with a low-intensity warm-up (like marching in place) and stretching period of five to ten minutes. The warm-up will prepare your heart for increased activity. The stretching will help you avoid tendon and muscle problems, which are common in people whose tendons have become brittle after years of high blood glucose levels.

After your warm-up and stretching, start the aerobic portion of your activity. One way to determine how rigorously you should exercise is by using a target heart rate zone. You'll want to keep your heart rate in this zone as you exercise. To determine your target heart rate zone, first subtract your age from 220. Multiply the resulting number first by 50 percent (or .5) to find the lower end of your target zone and then by 75 percent (or .75) to find the upper end of the zone. During exercise, count your heartbeats (by feeling the pulse on the inner side of your wrist) for six seconds and add a zero to the end of that

Easy Does It

You'll be less likely to experience problems if you increase your activity level slowly and gradually raise the duration and intensity.

number; that's the number of times your heart is beating per minute. You'll want that number to fall in the 50-75 percent range. If you find this intensity too taxing at first, try slowing your pace but increasing the length of time that you exercise.

18-117

Your Target Heart Rate

[220 – (your age)] × .5 to [220 - (your age)] × .75

Example: Target heart rate for a 54-year-old:

[220 - 54] × .5 to [220 - 54] × .75 = 83 to 125

Another way to assess your pace is with the "talk test": You want the exercise to get your heart pumping faster, but you never want to exercise so intensely that you can no longer comfortably carry on a conversation as you exercise.

Be sure to consult your diabetes care team for more specific advice regarding how often, how long, and how hard you should exercise.

It's always best to start your increase in physical activity slowly and build up gradually. If you find it uncomfortable to exercise near the higher range of your target zone, shoot for a lower intensity but a longer duration. As time passes, you'll be able to maintain a higher and higher level of activity for longer and longer periods of time.

Regardless of the activity you choose, you should end each activity period with ten minutes of cooldown and stretches. Slowly decrease your pace for several minutes rather than stopping abruptly. Then, take advantage of the fact that your muscles are warmed up to do some gentle stretching.

If you try to do some extra activity every other day, you will be amazed at the difference in your glucose control. Get moving every day and the benefits will be even greater.

PREEMPTING GLUCOSE PROBLEMS To avoid problems with your glucose levels during exercise, there are a number of things you can do:

1. Plan your activity to follow a meal so that it can help lower the blood glucose rise that follows eating.

2. Check your blood glucose 30 minutes before and then just prior to your activities. This way you can see which direction your glucose level is heading and anticipate a low in time to take preventive action.

3. If you are at risk for hypoglycemia, plan for possible hypoglycemia and carry glucose tablets with you in case symptoms of low blood glucose develop.

4. If you manage your diabetes with insulin, know the peak time of your insulin and plan your activities accordingly. You can help prevent possible hypoglycemia by avoiding exercise at the times when your insulin is peaking and therefore at its strongest.

5. When injecting insulin, avoid the muscle groups that you will be using during the activity. If you are a tennis player, for example, do not use your arm for your injection at the meal prior to your game. Most people find the abdomen or buttock to be a good injection site.

6. When planning to be extremely active, test your glucose prior to getting started. If your glucose level is near normal but you are at risk for hypoglycemia, you will need to eat prior to the activity. If you take insulin, you may need to lower your insulin dose or eat prior to the activity.

7. If your blood glucose before your activity is more than 250 mg/dl, check your urine for ketones. If they are present, activity will actually cause your blood glucose level to increase. An elevated glucose and positive ketones indicate that your diabetes is uncontrolled and you need to contact your health care team for advice immediately.

8. Monitor your glucose to see what effect activity has on you. Check it before exercise, every half hour during exercise, and when you are finished.

9. Be sure to drink plenty of fluids. Sweating means you are losing fluids that need to be replaced. Water is usually a great choice.

10. If during any activity you ever experience shortness of breath, chest pain, or leg cramps that go away with rest, contact your doctor immediately. These are all possible signs of blocked arteries and require an evaluation by your doctor.

11. If you repeatedly experience hypoglycemia during and/or after increased levels of activity, contact your doctor for a change in your medications.

The bottom line is: Being active needs to be fun. Your Mom never told you to go out and exercise with friends. She told you to go outside, have fun, and play. Play more, exercise less, and you will be surprised at how easy it is to get your muscles moving every day.

CHAPTER 9

Using Pills to Treat Diabetes

or many people with Type 2 diabetes, using food and activity to control blood glucose is not enough. For them, the new oral diabetes medications can be lifesavers—helping to lower their blood glucose and stave off diabetes complications.

Do Medications Mean I Have Failed?

Imagine yourself sailing down the interstate at 70 miles per hour. It is a flat, open road and you require a steady amount of fuel to keep you at this speed. Then you hit a mountain range. To continue at the same speed as you begin to ascend requires more and more fuel...you must press further down on the gas pedal to maintain a speed of 70 miles per hour. The disease of diabetes is similar in a way. When first diagnosed, you may be able to maintain a steady speed, or glucose range, with a few lifestyle modifications. However, the disease of diabetes has mountains built into its route—it is a progressive "uphill" disease that requires more and more "fuel" to keep your speed in your goal range.

In general, the first steps to take to return your glucose levels to as normal as possible are to increase the level of activity in your life and to change your relationship with food. Sometimes these steps can't lower your glucose levels enough to reach a normal range or, over time, they may not continue to keep your level within your goal range. You may then require medication to help you achieve or maintain your goal blood glucose levels. If and when this happens, do not look at the use of medications as a failure on your part in any way. Remember that diabetes is a chronic, progressive disease that requires more and more treatments over time to keep the blood glucose level under the same good control. Your goal, in the end, should not be to avoid medications but to avoid complications. Fortunately, recent years have seen the advent of several new and effective treatments that can help you reach that goal.

How Do Pills Work?

People with Type 1 diabetes make very little insulin, if any, so they are dependent on insulin injections to keep them healthy and well. Since the pills to treat diabetes are not the same as insulin and do not contain any insulin, they are of no use to people with Type 1 diabetes. The pills used to treat diabetes can lower blood glucose levels, but only in people with Type 2 diabetes, whose bodies still make some insulin but just don't use it well enough.

To understand the use of pills for the treatment of diabetes, you must first understand why your blood glucose levels are still high. For you and others with Type 2 diabetes, the problem in glucose control appears to be in no fewer than three areas. First, your muscles are not taking up the glucose in your bloodstream. Second, the liver is overproducing glucose, further increasing the glucose levels in your blood. And third, the insulin production by your pancreas cannot keep up with the high levels of glucose.

In this gradual system breakdown, the primary problem seems to be an insulin resistance in your muscles. Your muscles are not responding to your insulin and so the glucose is not being taken in by your muscles; instead, the glucose builds up in your blood. It's as if your cells are in their rooms, with the radio turned up very loud. Insulin and glucose are at the door, and insulin is knocking, but because the radio is up so loud, the cell cannot hear it.

The next problem lies in your liver. Your liver normally stops making glucose when it sees insulin. When you eat, your glucose level rises, which prompts the release of insulin from your pancreas. The insulin's job is to get the muscle cells to take in the glucose. When your liver sees the insulin, it knows that glucose has entered the system, so it stops releasing its own glucose stores. The insulin levels in your body normally decrease when your glucose levels drop, such as when you fast overnight or when it has been longer than four hours since you

> ## Help in a Pill
>
> Oral diabetes medications help the person with Type 2 diabetes make enough insulin to control glucose levels.

have eaten. Your liver does not see as much insulin, so it kicks into gear and begins to make glucose to keep your levels in a normal range. When you eat again and insulin is once again released, the liver detects the insulin and once again stops releasing its glucose stores. When your liver cells become insulin resistant, however, they cannot see the insulin released after a meal and they "think," wrongly, that your glucose levels are low. So your liver pumps out more glucose despite the fact that there's already glucose in the bloodstream waiting to get into your muscle cells.

The last and crucial problem is the inability of your pancreas, specifically the beta cells in your pancreas, to make enough insulin to keep up with this resistance. With progressive increases in glucose and fatty acids in your bloodstream and the excess demands to make more insulin, the beta cells are progressively poisoned and die off. When you reach a point where there are very few beta cells living, your blood glucose increases greatly, which further decreases the ability of the body to take up glucose, causing the elevated glucose levels seen in uncontrolled diabetes.

The actions of the pills available to treat the elevated glucose levels of diabetes work on these three problem areas. They stimulate your beta cells to make more insulin, they decrease your liver's glucose production, and they increase the sensitivity of your muscle cells to glucose. So, while most people with Type 2 diabetes still make some insulin, it is not enough to control glucose levels. The medications help your body make enough insulin available to control your glucose levels.

The oral diabetes medications available today fall into five different categories: sulfonylureas, biguanides, alpha-glucosidase inhibitors, thiazo-lidinediones, and meglitinides. The five types have different actions and support your body in different ways. As you and your health care providers begin to consider one or more of these pills to help keep your glucose levels in a healthy range, keep yourself completely informed. Know the names of all your medications, how much you need to take, and when to take them. Be aware of any possible side effects and whether or not drugs can be taken with any other medications you currently take. The following discussions can help you become familiar with the medications available.

Sulfonylureas

The sulfonylureas (sul-fa-nul-ur-ee-ahs) are the "original diabetes pill"; they were the first pills ever available to treat diabetes. Prior to their introduction, insulin was the only treatment for elevated glucose levels. Around the time of World War II, it was noticed that antibacterial agents called sulfa drugs also seemed to lower blood glucose. But it wasn't until the 1950s that this discovery would lead to the introduction in the United States of sulfalike medications, called sulfonylureas, for the treatment of diabetes.

Sulfonylureas work by stimulating your pancreas to release more insulin. The first medication that was available in this category is called Orinase

The Older Sulfonylureas in a Nutshell

BRAND NAME	GENERIC NAME	TYPICAL DAILY DOSE	MAXIMUM DOSE PER DAY	DURATION OF ACTION IN YOUR BODY
Orinase	tolbutamide	250–3,000 mg taken as a divided dose, twice a day	3,000 mg	6–12 hours
Tolinase	tolazamide	100–1,000 mg taken as a single or divided dose, once or twice a day	1,000 mg	24 hours
Diabinese	chlorpropamide	100–750 mg taken as a single dose, once a day	750 mg	24–72 hours

(its generic name is tolbutamide); it was followed shortly by Diabinese (chlorpropamide) and Tolinase (tolazamide). These medications are often referred to as "first generation sulfonylureas," since they were the first pills released in this category. Since the 1950s, newer and stronger sulfonylureas have become available. These include the "second generation sulfonylureas" Diabeta, Micronase, Glynase (all are brand names for the drug glyburide), and Glucotrol (glipizide) and, more recently, the "third generation sulfonylurea" Amaryl (glimepiride).

The sulfonylureas all operate by the same mechanism. They work on your beta cells, pushing them to make more insulin in order to lower your

The Newer Sulfonylureas in a Nutshell

BRAND NAME	GENERIC NAME	TYPICAL DAILY DOSE	MAXIMUM DOSE PER DAY	DURATION OF ACTION IN YOUR BODY
Micronase, Diabeta	glyburide	1.25–20 mg taken as a single or divided dose, once or twice a day	20 mg	24 hours
Glynase	micronized glyburide	1.5–6 mg taken as a single dose, once a day	6 mg	24 hours
Glucotrol	glipizide	5–20 mg taken as a single or divided dose, once or twice a day	20 mg	12–24 hours
Glucotrol XL	glipizide extended release	5–20 mg taken as a single dose, once a day	20 mg	24 hours
Amaryl	glimepiride	1–8 mg taken as a single or divided dose, once or twice a day	8 mg	24 hours

glucose level. Because of your insulin resistance, you require substantially more insulin than a non-insulin-resistant person to get the same amount of glucose into cells. In other words, your gas mileage has gone down. Instead of 20 miles for each gallon of gas, you now only get 10 miles to each gallon. It takes more gas to travel the same distance, just as it takes more insulin to keep your glucose levels normal.

These medications benefit you by lowering your glucose levels, but because they continually work on your pancreas, they cause insulin to be released even when it may not be needed. This is the major drawback, and causes the major side effect, of all the sulfonylurea medications; they can cause hypoglycemia, or low blood glucose (see Chapter 10 for more detailed information on hypoglycemia and how to treat it). Other side effects, although uncommon, include skin rashes, dark urine, stomach upset, and an increased sensitivity to the sun.

The first generation sulfonylurea Diabinese, with its very prolonged duration of action in the body, carries a greater risk of prolonged and severe hypoglycemia under certain conditions. Diabinese can also cause additional side effects including hyponatremia (a low level of sodium in the blood) and a flushing of your skin when you ingest alcohol.

Sulfonylureas are taken daily, at the same time each day, generally about 30 minutes before your meal. If taken just once a day, they are usually taken with your first meal of the day. Because these medications are broken down by the liver and then eventually leave your body through your urine (via your kidneys), these medications should be used with caution if you have kidney or liver disease. In these diseases, the route by which the medication is broken down or leaves your body may be blocked, which can cause the medicine to accumulate in your body and cause very prolonged hypoglycemia.

Your sulfonylurea is working properly if your blood glucose values remain in a healthy range and you do not suffer from any episodes of hypoglycemia. Check your blood glucose often, both before and after meals, especially if this is a new medication for you or your medication dose has recently been changed. Pay particularly close attention to your glucose readings before your midday and evening meals. Another clue that your medication is working is having a HbA1c level below seven percent and blood glucose levels in a healthy range most of the time. If they're not, review your activity and eating patterns, ask yourself if you are missing medication doses, and see if there is any pattern to your high or low glucose levels. If your numbers remain too high or too low or you are not

> ### Even Better
>
> Newer, stronger versions of sulfonylureas, the original "diabetes pills," continue to be important weapons in the fight to control blood glucose in Type 2 diabetes.

satisfied with your control, your doctor may need to change your dose or even switch you to a different medication.

Biguanides

Biguanides (bi-gwan-ides) are the second type of diabetes medication. The current and only biguanide available in the United States is Glucophage, also known by its generic name, metformin. In the 1960s, a precursor of metformin, DBI-TD (also known as phenformin), was introduced as a twice-a-day medication for the control of glucose levels. It was a very effective medication, but it was removed from the market because of a rare but fatal complication called lactic acidosis. Lactic acidosis is a condition in which lactic acids build up in the bloodstream; it is fatal in 50 percent of the people who develop the condition. This devastating side effect prompted researchers to develop metformin, a safer version of DBI-TD. It was introduced in Europe about 40 years ago but it was not available in the United States until 1995.

How Glucophage works is not yet completely understood. Its major action is to cause the liver to produce less glucose and fewer triglycerides. Since Glucophage does not directly affect insulin levels and probably does not affect the uptake of glucose by your muscles, it is not very effective for controlling post-meal glucose levels. Its greatest benefit seems to be in decreasing the output of glucose by your liver during periods when you are fasting (such as between meals or at night).

When it has been more than four hours since you have eaten, your insulin levels have generally dropped, as have your blood glucose levels. As a result, the liver normally steps up its production of glucose. However, if you are insulin resistant, your liver doesn't seem to see insulin even when there is plenty in the bloodstream (such as after a meal) and mistakenly acts as if your blood glucose is low. It makes glucose that it releases into your bloodstream—even though your blood glucose levels are already high. Glucophage stops this excess glucose production by the liver.

Since the most extended period of fasting for many people occurs overnight, the liver tends to be very busy during that time. As a result, the morning glucose levels tend to be the highest of the day. Glucophage works well to prevent these early-morning highs by decreasing glucose production while you sleep. In addition, it seems to be effective in lowering triglycerides and LDL cholesterol levels. As an added benefit, it appears to cause less weight gain than most of the other diabetic medications and does not cause hypoglycemia. With all of these positives, it is not surprising that Glucophage is currently the most commonly prescribed diabetic medication in the United States.

These accolades aside, the side effects of Glucophage mar its sparkling reputation. About 30 percent of the people who take Glucophage develop stomach upset or diarrhea; about 3 percent of those individuals find these side effects so intolerable that they cannot continue the medication. However, if your dose of Glucophage starts out low and is slowly increased over time and if you take the medicine with or immediately after you have eaten, these symptoms can be minimized or eliminated. Sometimes decreasing the total dose or only taking the medication with the evening meal can eliminate the side effects. If, after trying these adjustments, you are still plagued by diarrhea, loose stools, or frequent or uncontrollable bowel movements, talk to your doctor. Such side effects can obviously decrease your quality of life and you need not tolerate them, since there are other medications available to help you achieve glucose control.

Like its predecessor, Glucophage can cause lactic acidosis, but this is extremely rare; only about 30 out of every million people who take the medication experience it each year. The signs and symptoms of lactic acidosis are unusual muscle pain, fast and shallow breathing, slow or unsteady heartbeat, vomiting, or a serious infection accompanied by dehydration and fever. In order to avoid this potentially dangerous side effect, there are a few precautions that need to be taken by anyone on this medication:

- Glucophage should never be used by anyone who drinks in excess or is a binge drinker.
- It should not be taken by anyone who has liver or kidney disease.
- It should not be taken by anyone who has a condition, such as heart failure, that results in poor circulation or a condition, such as serious lung disease, that causes low oxygen states.
- In general, Glucophage is not prescribed for people more than 80 years of age unless their kidney and liver function are tested, frequently monitored, and found to be normal.
- Precaution must also be taken by anyone who requires any type of medical test involving injection of a contrast dye. During such dye tests, the kidney excretion of lactic acid is slowed, which can allow the

Watch Out for Glucophage If You Have These Conditions

Kidney Failure

The creatinine level in your blood is a measurement of your kidney function. For women, this level should be less than 1.4 mg/dl and for men less than 1.5 mg/dl. If your creatinine level is greater than this, you should not be taking Glucophage.

Lung or Heart Disease

Examples include severe asthma and congestive heart failure.

Liver Disease

Hepatitis is one example. ALT is a measure of an enzyme present in your liver. When your liver is irritated or diseased, this enzyme becomes elevated.

Heavy Alcohol Intake or Binge Drinking

Heavy intake is considered to be more than 2-3 drinks per day (a drink is 4 ounces of wine, 12 ounces of beer, or 1½ ounces of hard liquor).

Advanced Age

As we age, our kidney function naturally decreases. After age 80, blood creatinine levels are no longer the best indicator of kidney function. Kidney function is best evaluated by a 24-hour measurement of your creatinine clearance, which requires you to collect your urine for 24 hours straight so that your kidney function can be checked.

Contrast-Dye Studies

You will need to temporarily stop taking Glucophage. Have your kidney function reevaluated before you restart the medication.

acid to build up in the blood. If you need to have such a test, you will need to stop taking Glucophage before the test and not start taking it again for two to three days afterward. But do not stop taking Glucophage unless directed by your doctor. Consult your doctor first.

Glucophage comes in 500, 850, and 1,000 mg tablets. It is generally taken twice a day, once in the morning and once at night. Occasionally, due to side effects, it is taken either just once a day in the evening or in smaller doses, before each meal, three times a day. The initial daily dose is usually 500 mg with your evening meal. The daily dose is then increased by 500 mg each week until the usual, maximum dose of 2,000 mg per day is reached. This is generally taken as 1,000 mg, twice a day. Above 2,000 mg per day, there appears to be little added benefit, and additional side effects are likely. If for any reason you must stop taking Glucophage for more than three days, you may find that you have to restart at the 500 mg dose in order to avoid side effects. Most people who have to stop the medication for three days for a contrast-dye study are able to restart the medication at their usual dose without experiencing significant side effects.

Alpha-Glucosidase Inhibitors (AGIs)

Alpha-glucosidase (glue-kos-a-dase) inhibitors, or AGIs, are the third type of pill available to treat diabetes. There are two medications available in the United States that fall into this class: Precose (acarbose) and Glyset (miglitol). Both medications work on your small intestines, where starches and large sugar molecules are broken down and absorbed.

One of the primary enzymes that allows for the absorption of glucose into your blood is alpha-glucosidase. This enzyme is in the lining of your small intestines, and its effectiveness is partially blocked by these medications. As a result, glucose is more slowly absorbed, and some glucose may not be absorbed at all but rather digested by bacteria found further downstream in your intestines. This delay in the absorption of glucose into the blood helps to prevent the sudden surges of glucose that can occur after eating. While these medications do not appear to cause weight loss, they do moderately lower the blood glucose level after meals and very mildly lower glucose levels in the fasting state, such as first thing in the morning.

When AGIs are used, not all of your food is absorbed, so it has ample time to react with the

bacteria and yeast normally found in your bowels.
These bacteria and yeast break down starches
and sugars to gases. This results in the main side
effects reported with these medicines—diarrhea
and the tremendous production of gas. About 80
percent of all people who use an AGI experience
these side effects, and
a number of those
people find they
cannot tolerate these
effects in the long
term. Other side
effects are more rare
and include liver

> ### AGI Got It
>
> AGIs cause a delay in the
> absorption of glucose
> into the blood, which
> helps prevent the sudden
> surge of glucose that can
> occur after you eat.

irritation, so these medications should not be used
if you have liver disease. In addition, like
Glucophage, the AGIs can build up in your system
if your kidneys are not functioning well. If your
creatinine level is currently above—or *ever*
exceeds—2 mg/dl you should not take these medications.

AGIs used alone cannot cause hypoglycemia.
However, caution is required if they are taken
with a medication, such as sulfonylureas, which
can cause low blood glucose levels. Because the
AGIs delay the absorption of certain sugars, the
hypoglycemia can only be treated with glucose

tablets, milk, corn syrup, honey, or fruit juices. The absorption of any other starches or sugars would be delayed, resulting in more prolonged hypoglycemia.

The usual dose of AGIs is 25 to 100 mg per meal taken no more than three times a day. Any dosage increases should be done very slowly, about once every other week to once each month. The slow increase in dose may help to decrease the potential side effects as much as possible and help the body become accustomed to the changes these medications cause.

With their minimal effectiveness and frequent side effects, the class of AGIs has not been extremely popular with people in the United States who have diabetes. Oddly enough, however, they are the number-one prescribed diabetes medication in Germany.

Thiozolidinediones ("Glitazones")

Thiozolidinediones (thigh-ah-zo-la-deen-die-owns), commonly referred to as "glitazones," are the fourth, and most controversial, group of medications available to treat diabetes. Also known as TZDs or insulin sensitizers, they ushered in a new age in the treatment of Type 2 diabetes when they were first introduced in 1997. For the first time ever, a medication was available to treat and decrease the main problem of Type 2 diabetes—insulin resistance. The glitazones work on the genes inside your fat cells and may work elsewhere in the body as well. They start by stimulating a molecule called PPAR gamma, and this stimulation has several results. PPAR gamma causes your fat cells to take up more fatty acids and glucose, leaving fewer fatty acids for your muscle cells. The muscle cells then turn back to using glucose as their preferred fuel source and consequently increase their sensitivity to insulin. This is significant since the muscles normally take up 80 percent of the glucose from a meal.

A similar change occurs in your liver. As your insulin resistance decreases, your liver begins to make less glucose, because it can once again easily "see" the insulin in your bloodstream. Significant changes happen in the beta cells of your pancreas, too. First, the drop in your glucose and fatty acid levels result in lower insulin levels in your blood. This drop, coupled with what appears to be a direct protective effect that the glitazones have on the beta cells, benefits your beta cells to such an extent that they are able to recover from the stress of diabetes and Syndrome X and live much longer. So the glitazones may actually prevent the downhill slide that eventually leads to the inability of your pancreas to secrete insulin and the subsequent need for insulin injections. And the benefits don't end there.

The glitazones have been shown to have a protective effect on the blood vessels of your body. Consequently, they reduce the holes in the blood vessels of the kidneys through which albumin is lost. So they may play a direct role in preventing diabetic kidney disease. Studies have also shown that the glitazones improve the condition of your coronary arteries (the blood vessels that feed the heart), not just indirectly by lowering blood fats, but directly. Likewise, when you take glitazones, your level of beneficial HDL cholesterol increases, your triglyceride level drops, your blood pressure decreases, and your clotting factors improve, all of which decrease your risk of coronary heart disease.

Unfortunately, controversy has surrounded the glitazones since 1999, when Rezulin (troglitazone), the first in this class of medications, made headline news. The news was not good. The early clinical trials of Rezulin had shown that liver irritation occurs about three times more commonly in people using the medication versus those not taking it. After Rezulin hit the market in 1997, case reports of liver failure and death began to trickle into the U.S. Food & Drug Administration (FDA). Still, the cases appeared to be very rare. At the time, Rezulin was the only glitazone on the market, and more than a million people were successfully managing their diabetes with it. Indeed, it was proving itself to be a very valuable medication. So the FDA mandated that Rezulin could continue to be prescribed but only with more closely monitored liver function testing.

As the liver side effects of Rezulin continued to make news throughout 1999 and early 2000, two new medications in this class hit the market. They were Actos (pioglitazone) and Avandia (rosiglitazone). These two new medications lacked evidence of the serious liver side effects of Rezulin. So the makers of Rezulin stopped making the medication and removed it from the market in March 2000. Today, literally millions of patients have taken the two new medicines with no evidence of liver complications or side effects any greater than those observed in clinical trials. The new glitazones promise to show the similar, beneficial effects common to all glitazones, with some minor differences.

Very limited and preliminary studies have suggested differences between Avandia and Actos; these differences can play a role in your doctor's choice of medication for you. Actos appears to be more beneficial in improving lipid levels than Avandia. But Actos may be associated with more weight gain than Avandia. This weight gain occurs in about 30 percent of those who take Actos, although it does not appear to have a harmful effect on blood pressure or lipid levels.

The side effects of these agents to date appear to be very few and, oddly enough, related to their beneficial effects in your body. Weight gain, possible increased risk of hypoglycemia if combined with other specific types of diabetes medications, an increased risk of pregnancy, anemia, edema, and liver irritation are possible side effects of both Actos and Avandia.

Why the glitazones cause weight gain is not entirely understood, but it could occur for several reasons. Weight increase is not an uncommon side effect for any medication that improves diabetes control. As your blood glucose levels

The Current "Glitazone" Lineup

TRADE NAME	GENERIC NAME	STRENGTHS	DOSE	MAXIMUM DOSE
Avandia	rosiglitazone	2, 4, and 8 mg	once or twice a day	8 mg
Actos	pioglitazone	15, 30, and 45 mg	once a day	45 mg

improve, your body is now able to use the glucose for energy or to save it for future use, instead of losing the glucose through the urine. You are now holding on to the fuel you take in, so if you take in more fuel than you need, your "storage tanks" become that much more visible.

Another common reason for weight gain from diabetes treatment is the food intake required to correct frequent hypoglycemia. Although the glitazones do not cause hypoglycemia when they are taken alone, combining them with a sulfonylurea, a meglitinide, or insulin can result in hypoglycemia. The glitazones decrease your insulin resistance, which allows the other medications to work too well, causing you to increase your food intake to keep up with the insulin output they cause. By simply decreasing, or even eliminating, the amount of sulfonylurea, meglitinide, or insulin, the hypoglycemia diminishes, as does the weight gain. You should not significantly decrease the dose or eliminate any medication, however, without prior approval from your diabetes care team.

Some weight gain is caused by fluid retention. The fluid retention is due to a relaxing of your blood vessels, which were previously constricted due to your high insulin levels. This is a good thing for your health, but the extra capacity created by the expansion of your blood vessels is filled with salt and water. The fluid buildup can lead to edema and can also cause a dilution of your red blood cells, resulting in a mild "anemia" that is probably not of real concern. The water retention appears as an increase in your weight, as well as swelling, especially around your feet and ankles. The side effect of edema causes about five percent of those who take glitazones to discontinue the medication. In addition, if you currently have a serious level of congestive heart failure, the extra fluid may cause shortness of breath and a worsening of your condition. For this reason, the glitazones should not be used in people with severe congestive heart failure.

An increased risk of pregnancy occurs for two different reasons. First, the glitazones decrease the effectiveness of birth control pills, which makes this method of birth control less effective in preventing pregnancy. Using an alternative method of birth control generally solves this problem. Second, the increased risk of pregnancy is a direct result of the glitazones' ability to decrease insulin resistance. Polycystic ovary syndrome (POS) is a condition caused by high levels of insulin and is characterized by a lack of menstruation and infertility. Glitazones decrease the insulin resistance, decrease the levels of circulating insulin, and cause the ovaries to decrease the production of male hormones, which allows the menstrual cycle to resume and fertility to return.

Because Avandia and Actos are related to Rezulin, they carry with them the legacy of the Rezulin liver complications. The FDA has required that liver monitoring be done every two months during the first year of glitazone use and periodically thereafter. While this required level of monitoring is 50 percent less frequent than that which was required for Rezulin, the political heat on these newer medicines is so hot that it is doubtful that this requirement will be removed, even though no significant liver complications have been reported.

The time it takes for the glitazones to become effective in your system is considerably longer than for most diabetes medications, which can begin lowering glucose levels within hours of their ingestion. Because the glitazones work on a cellular level, through your genes, the decrease in insulin resistance and subsequent lower glucose levels are very slow to occur. The converse is true in that the effect is also very slow to disappear. It can take up to four months for you to see the full effect of a glitazone on your glucose levels, but usually some effect can been seen in the first one to two weeks. Because of this slow pace, increasing the dose of glitazones is usually done only after waiting four to six weeks to see what effect they have had on your levels.

Meglitinides

Meglitinides (ma-glit-tin-eyeds) are the newest and the fifth type of medication available to treat Type 2 diabetes. This class of medications first became available in 1998 with the release of Prandin (repaglinide). Meglitinides, which are similar to sulfonylureas, stimulate insulin release by the beta cells of your pancreas to help lower rising glucose levels. However, they differ from the sulfonylureas in that they are much shorter-acting and begin working very quickly to increase your insulin level while your food is being digested and glucose is entering your bloodstream. In addition to acting quickly, they also leave your bloodstream quickly, so your body doesn't keep releasing insulin beyond when it's needed, thus reducing your risk of hypoglycemia.

Sulfonylureas are generally taken just once a day and cause a steady release of insulin throughout the day, whether you eat or not. Meglitinides are different because they are taken just before meals. And because they work very quickly, they allow you to vary the timing and frequency of your meals each day. You take this medication one, two, three, or four times a day, depending on how many meals you eat. If you need or want to miss a meal, you skip that pill entirely.

Prandin comes in 0.5, 1, and 2 mg doses. The total daily dose should not exceed 16 mg. Because it does cause your pancreas to release insulin, Prandin has the potential to cause hypoglycemia, especially if you take your pill but your meal is unexpectedly delayed or if you end up eating significantly less than you usually do. However, the risk of hypoglycemia is less than that with the sulfonylureas because Prandin is a much shorter-acting medication and therefore does not remain in your system for extended periods after the meal. Other side effects or symptoms that have been reported with Prandin use include cold- and flu-like symptoms, diarrhea, joint aches, and back pain. In addition, a rash and stomach upset can occur, but they are also quite rare.

The benefit of the meglitinides, when compared to sulfonylureas, is that they do not contain a sulfur group and thus, do not cause sulfa allergies. In addition, to date, Prandin is the only medication that can be used safely by people who have kidney and liver problems, as it does not significantly affect these conditions in an adverse way. Nonetheless, they must still be used with caution and continual monitoring.

Prandin was recently joined by another meglitinide, nateglinide (Starlix), which was approved by the FDA in December 2000. It has a very rapid onset of action, releasing insulin quickly, but has a short duration of action, so high insulin levels are short-lived. Starlix comes in two strengths, 60 mg and 120 mg. Like Prandin, it will be taken just before each meal. It looks like the benefits of this new medication will include an even lower risk of hypoglycemia and the lack of need for a trial period to determine the proper dose (which is necessary with Prandin).

New Treatments on the Horizon

Glucagonlike peptide 1 (GLP-1) is another promising-looking treatment. GLP-1 is a naturally occurring, proteinlike substance found in our intestines. When released, it stimulates insulin secretion, slows the intestinal absorption of glucose, and reduces appetite. In other words, it does exactly what you'd want a treatment for Type 2 diabetes to do. Unfortunately, in its current form, it is broken down in a few minutes. Research into this exciting peptide continues and is centering on oral medications that will stop the breakdown. Expect to hear more about this in the coming years.

New glitazones are also in the pipeline. Some are more potent, significantly improving lipid levels and actually causing weight loss. In addition, research involving the newest potential diabetes medication looks extremely promising. These drawing-board medications do not look or act anything like the drugs that are currently available. But they have a profound effect on cholesterol, lowering it by 80 percent, and they decrease glucose levels, all without any apparent side effects, at least in rats.

The drug treatments available to the person with Type 2 diabetes have never been so plentiful—or so effective. The boom in diabetes treatments during the last few years has been so significant that for the first time people can be told that diabetes complications are no longer a given and that achieving absolutely normal glucose control, without hypoglycemia, is an absolute possibility.

CHAPTER 10

Hypoglycemia

Diabetes management focuses on lowering high blood glucose, but there's a potential side effect called a hypoglycemic reaction that can be equally dangerous. Especially for people who have had diabetes for a long time or who take certain medications or insulin, being able to recognize and treat it is a basic skill for their diabetes toolbox.

Strange Happenings

It's 5:00 P.M.: You test your blood glucose and take your diabetes medication. You start to eat your dinner but, midway through, the phone rings, taking you away from the meal. By the time you return, the food is cold and you decide not to finish what's left on your plate. All is fine until a few hours later, when you start to feel dizzy and nauseous, begin sweating, and notice that your heart is beating very fast and hard. You test your blood glucose—the meter reads 52 mg/dl! You grab some orange juice, a few cookies, and a handful of grapes. You start feeling a bit better, and by the time you finish a glass of milk and a turkey sandwich, you're on solid ground and everything is back to normal. You check your glucose again before heading to bed and are shocked to find a reading of 269 mg/dl. What the heck is going on?

In two words, you experienced a *hypoglycemic reaction*. The high blood glucose level that followed, called a food rebound, resulted from the lifesaving steps you took to increase your blood glucose.

What Is Hypoglycemia?

As its name suggests, hypoglycemia means low blood sugar (*hypo* means low and *glycemia* means glucose). It's sometimes referred to as an "insulin reaction," a "low," "insulin shock," or just plain "shock." No matter the term used, hypoglycemia is one of the most common, and most dangerous, side effects of blood-glucose-lowering medication.

For the person with diabetes, the goal of treatment is to lower glucose levels to as close to normal as possible. If the treatment to obtain this goal contains insulin and/or one of the insulin-

Symptoms of Hypoglycemia

The onset of symptoms is generally sudden.

EARLY SYMPTOMS	LATE SYMPTOMS
(caused by the release of epinephrine and decreasing blood glucose levels)	(caused by the decreasing availability of glucose to your brain)
Dizziness	Headache
Pale or flushed face	Blurred vision
Irritability	Slurred speech
Hunger	Confusion
Sweating	Euphoria
Rapid heartbeat	Hostility
Fatigue or weakness	Lack of coordination
Nervousness or anxiousness	Drowsiness
Shakiness	Convulsions
Queasiness	Loss of consciousness

stimulating medications (a sulfonylurea or Prandin), then hypoglycemia is a risk. Hypoglycemia can occur if you take too much insulin or too large a dose of medication, miss or delay a meal, eat too little food for the amount of insulin or pills you have taken, increase your normal level of activity, drink alcohol, or any combination of these factors.

As stated previously, the normal range for blood glucose is 70 to 110 mg/dl on a plasma-calibrated meter or 60 to 100 mg/dl on a whole-blood meter.

If your blood glucose falls below this level, you're in trouble. Your brain and nervous system, remember, depend solely on glucose for energy. To try to raise the glucose level, your brain sends out emergency signals. As a result, your alpha cells, located in your pancreas, release glucagon. The glucagon signals your liver and your muscles to release stored glycogen and change it back to glucose in an attempt to raise your blood glucose level to a normal range. Meanwhile, the release of the hormone epinephrine increases your hunger and causes a resistance to insulin's action. Other hormones, cortisol and growth hormone, are also released to counteract insulin and raise your blood glucose levels.

Outwardly, you may begin to feel dizzy, hungry, sick to your stomach, shaky, or very

Warning!

Hypoglycemia is a risk if you are on insulin or insulin-stimulating medications such as a sulfonylurea or Prandin.

fatigued and weak. You may notice that you are sweaty, your heart is beating fast, your face is pale or flushed, or your mouth and lips are tingling or numb. These early signs of low blood glucose are primarily caused by the release of epinephrine.

If the glucose continues to drop, less and less is available to your brain. You may develop a headache, blurred vision, slurred speech, and confusion. You may become quite uncoordinated, and your general state of mind can be either euphoric or quite hostile and belligerent. If the low glucose level continues, you can lose consciousness, have a seizure, and possibly lapse into a coma. Hypoglycemia can even result in death.

So, hypoglycemia happens when your blood glucose level drops too low and there is not enough energy to keep your body—and especially your brain—functioning adequately. Your gas tank is empty, the fuel warning light is on, and you are driving on fumes. If you don't get gas soon, you will be stalled on the side of the road, going nowhere.

What Do I Do About It?

The best time to treat hypoglycemia is as soon as you recognize the first symptoms. Do not wait! Food is the best remedy for hypoglycemia, but not just any food. You want something that will get in there fast and raise your glucose levels. While a chocolate bar may seem like a wonderful choice, it actually takes quite a bit of time for it to raise your glucose levels. The sucrose from the granulated sugar starts the process, but the fat and protein in the chocolate bar take much more time to break down, delaying the rise in glucose. You want something fast, something that works immediately to raise your glucose levels. Simple carbohydrates and liquid carbohydrates fit this bill. Glucose tablets, sugar cubes, fruit juice, milk, and hard candies are your best bet. They are absorbed quickly into your bloodstream and begin raising glucose levels within five to ten minutes.

Untreated hypoglycemia or a delay in treating a low blood glucose level can result in a severe hypoglycemic reaction in which you are unable to swallow liquids or food and may even become unconscious. Anyone who takes insulin to manage their diabetes is most at risk for this type of reaction. Others at risk for severe hypoglycemia are those who have had diabetes a long time and have developed hypoglycemia unawareness, in which they have difficulty recognizing the symptoms of low blood sugar until it is too late and they are unable to help themselves.

For anyone who takes insulin and anyone with hypoglycemia unawareness, an additional safety net, a glucagon emergency kit, needs to be kept on hand for emergencies. Glucagon is an injection that is given to the person having the severe reaction. This injected glucagon is a synthetic version of the hormone found in the alpha cells of the pancreas, the hormone that signals the liver and muscles to release stored glycogen. Anyone

How to Treat a Low Blood Glucose Level

1. Check your blood glucose (but ONLY if possible).
2. If you are in doubt and unable to check your blood glucose, ALWAYS assume that your glucose level is low.
3. Eat 15 grams of a fast-acting carbohydrate. That's equal to any of the following:
   - 3–4 glucose tabs
   - 4 ounces of fruit juice
   - 5 sugar cubes
   - 1 small box of raisins
   - 1 cup of skim milk
   - 1 tablespoon of honey
   - 6 hard candies
4. Wait 15 minutes, then check your blood glucose level again.
5. If symptoms are still present or blood sugar is less than 70, repeat step 3.
6. **IF THE PERSON IS UNABLE TO SWALLOW OR IS UNCONSCIOUS, A GLUCAGON INJECTION MUST BE GIVEN!** This should be done even if you are unsure that the blood sugar is low.
7. If symptoms are gone and it is more than one hour from a mealtime, eat a small snack that includes a protein, a fat, and a carbohydrate, such as a turkey sandwich with mayonnaise.
8. Call your doctor if you experience frequent or severe hypoglycemic reactions.

at severe risk of hypoglycemia should have a *glucagon emergency kit* and needs to train those around them how to use it. The kit is available, with a doctor's prescription, at pharmacies.

If you take insulin or an insulin-stimulating medication, you can reduce your risk of hypoglycemia. It's all a matter of education and preparation. Be sure to check your blood glucose levels frequently. Anticipate the situations that may trigger hypoglycemia (such as not eating enough at mealtime, as in our opening example) and take steps to adjust; plan ahead for increased activity or changes in your routine. Learn how to recognize and treat symptoms of low blood glucose, and stash sugar *everywhere*. Wear identification that states that you have diabetes. Teach your friends and family how to recognize the symptoms of low blood glucose and how to help if you hit a low. And if you take insulin, make sure those around you know how to treat you in case of an emergency and know where you keep your glucagon emergency kit.

Be Prepared!

Anyone who is at severe risk of developing hypoglycemia should have a glucagon emergency kit and should train those around them how and when to use it.

CHAPTER 11

Insulin

As unpleasant as the thought of having to give yourself a shot might be, it cannot compare to the devastating long-term complications that result from uncontrolled diabetes. Besides, the future of insulin therapy is looking pain-free!

Sticking to Control

Mention the word insulin and just about everyone has a story, and it generally doesn't have a happy ending. "My Aunt Grace started insulin and, shortly after, she went blind." "I know this guy, he takes insulin and he's always sick." "My friend had to start insulin and she's gained 40 pounds over the last year!" In addition to personal tales like this, health care professionals have been known to threaten their patients with insulin as a motivational tool. The person is told that "if you don't get it together, take your pills, strictly follow your diet, and exercise, I'll have to resort to insulin to manage your diabetes" or "if you fail this, all we will have left is insulin."

For these reasons, and the simple fact that very few of us relish the thought of willingly sticking a needle into our skin, insulin has always been viewed as the end of the line, where no other hope exists. This is not true. To understand your possible need for insulin, you need to remember the chronic, progressive nature of diabetes; you need to remember that the enemy is not insulin, but rather uncontrolled glucose levels; and you need to keep your eye on the goal: a complication-free life.

As has been mentioned, diabetes is a chronic disease that takes progressively more and more action to maintain glucose levels in a healthy range. You might first start out with just dietary changes and increased activity in your life; then you need a pill; then two pills; then a handful of pills; and finally a handful of pills and insulin—all to keep your glucose levels within your goal range. Because of the progressive nature of diabetes, if you live long enough, you will need insulin. Some need it sooner than others. You might need to live to be 137 before your time would come, but given what we know about diabetes today and the treatments we currently have available, you will eventually need insulin.

People often state that "I will do anything to get this diabetes under control, but I will never take insulin." Insulin is viewed as the ultimate and final failure. You have lost control and there is no other hope. You now have the "bad" diabetes. You now have the "serious type" of diabetes. The reality is that there are really only two types of diabetes, either *controlled* diabetes or *uncontrolled* diabetes, and you want to be in the controlled, uncomplicated group. What medications you take to maintain your glucose levels, how often you test your glucose levels, and how dedicated you are to your self-care in no way indicate good or bad, failure or success. *All* diabetes is serious, regardless of what type you have. Commit yourself to doing whatever it takes to keep yourself healthy. Elevated glucose levels result in complications, and if you need to inject insulin to prevent them, do it!

The First Diabetes Treatment

On January 23, 1922, at the University of Toronto, Dr. Frederick G. Banting and his student, C.H. Best, made one of the greatest discoveries of the twentieth century. They successfully treated a human diabetic with insulin, ending the death sentence for people suffering from diabetes. Prior to that discovery, there was no treatment for diabetes. Those with Type 1 died very quickly, while those with Type 2 died more slowly, suffering horrible complications prior to death. The University of Toronto immediately gave pharmaceutical companies license to produce insulin free of all royalties. In early 1923, about one year after the first test injection, insulin became widely available when Eli Lilly and Company marketed Iletin, the first commercially available insulin, which was extracted from the pancreata of stockyard animals.

Animal insulin worked well on the whole, saving millions of lives, but it was not an exact match with the human hor-

Reprieved

The successful treatment of a human with the insulin from an animal ended the death sentence that came with a diagnosis of diabetes.

mone and sometimes caused side effects such as skin rashes and allergic reactions that resulted in a loss of tissue at the injection sites. For the next 60 years, insulin would be one of the most studied proteins in the world. During this time, people with diabetes relied on a hormone purified from animals, primarily cattle and pigs.

In 1978, a fledgling biotechnology company named Genentech produced the first synthetically manufactured insulin that could be made in large amounts. Using bacteria or yeast as miniature "factories," the gene for human insulin was inserted into the bacterial DNA. The result was human insulin, called recombinant DNA insulin, which did not cause the problems that animal insulin sometimes caused. This new insulin, called Humulin, changed the treatment of diabetes when it became widely available in the early 1980s. Today, almost all people with diabetes who require insulin use a type of recombinant human insulin rather than animal insulin.

One Type Does Not Fit All

If you need insulin, the decision to take it is a good one. One thing that we know about insulin is that it always works. It will lower your glucose levels when taken correctly, in the proper amount and at the proper times.

As discussed previously, insulin is a small protein-like molecule made by the beta cells in the pancreas. Its major action is to provide your muscle and fat cells with glucose and tell your liver to make less glucose. If you have Type 1 diabetes, you are *insulin dependent*, as you depend on insulin injections to live. Your pancreas does not make enough insulin, if it makes any at all, to maintain your body's functions. If you have Type 2 diabetes, you may be *insulin requiring*; you may require insulin to supplement what your pancreas makes in order to maintain your body's functions.

There are different kinds of insulin, all with different characteristics. When determining the best insulin for you, there are three important characteristics to understand and consider. The first is the *onset* of the insulin. This is the length of time it takes the insulin to reach your bloodstream and begin to lower your glucose level. Next is the *peak time* of the insulin. This is the time when your insulin is at its maximum strength in terms of lowering your glucose level. The last characteristic of insulin to consider is its *duration*. This is the length of time that insulin remains in your body, continuing to lower your glucose levels.

With an understanding of the characteristics of insulin, you and your health care team have five (soon to be six) different types of insulin to consider. Very often these insulins will be used in some sort of combination in order to meet your required onset, peak-time, and duration needs. And while the characteristics of insulin types have been studied and documented at length, you need to understand that there is a uniqueness to each of us and that your response to insulin may vary from what is predicted. For this reason, taking complete, detailed notes of your glucose testing results, the timing of your tests, and your insulin injections becomes vitally important to understanding how insulin works in your body specifically.

The Types, Your Choices

When insulin first became available in 1923, there was only one type, *regular insulin*. While it was animal-based back then, it is still available today in a recombinant DNA form. Regular insulin, also called R insulin, is a short-acting insulin that usually begins working within 30 to 60 minutes, peaks two to four hours after injection, and is usually gone in six to eight hours.

In the early days of insulin therapy, the needles that were used to inject insulin were thick and needed to be sharpened by hand with a honing stone or razor strap before each use. The syringes were glass and needed to be boiled and cleaned every day. The pain and inconvenience of this created a drive to develop an insulin that was longer-acting so that fewer injections were needed. In the 1950s, European researchers developed two new insulin preparations that cut the required four to six injections a day down to two.

The first of these new insulin preparations was *NPH insulin*, which added a fish protein, protamine, to regular insulin to retard its absorption. NPH is an intermediate-acting insulin that gener-

Activity of the Various Insulin Types Available Today

TYPE OF INSULIN	ONSET	PEAK	DURATION	LOW BLOOD GLUCOSE MOST LIKELY TO OCCUR
Rapid-Acting				
lispro	5–10 minutes	1–2 hours	3–5 hours	2–3 hours
Short-Acting				
regular	30–60 minutes	2–4 hours	6–8 hours	3–5 hours
Intermediate-Acting				
NPH	2–4 hours	6–10 hours	16–24 hours	6–12 hours
Lente	3–4 hours	6–12 hours	20–26 hours	7–14 hours
Long-Acting				
Ultralente	4–6 hours	10–20 hours	24–36 hours	12–24 hours
Premixed				
70/30	30–60 minutes	2 & 8 hours	16–24 hours	3 & 9 hours
50/50	30–60 minutes	2 & 8 hours	16–24 hours	3 & 9 hours
75/25	5–10 minutes	1 & 8 hours	16–24 hours	2 & 9 hours

Remember, onset, peak, and duration times are all approximate. Each person is different and each will have a unique response time to insulin.

ally starts working in two to four hours, peaks in six to ten hours, and is gone from the system in 16 to 24 hours.

The other new preparation yielded two insulin types, *Lente* and *Ultralente* insulin. These insulins were made by crystallizing regular insulin to different degrees. By crystallizing the insulin, it took longer for the insulin to be absorbed, thus prolonging its action in the body. Lente insulin, an intermediate-acting insulin like NPH, generally starts working in three to four hours, peaks in 6 to 12 hours, and lasts for 20 to 26 hours.

By comparison, Ultralente is crystallized to a greater extent and is considered a long-acting insulin due to its length of duration in the body. It generally starts working in 4 to 6 hours, has a peak action at 10 to 20 hours, and is usually gone from the body 24 to 36 hours after the injection. Because of its extended length of action, it is often referred to as a "peakless" insulin, with a seemingly continuous release over a very long period of time. However, studies have shown that Ultralente insulin is absorbed at different rates in different people and does "peak," but not in a predictable manner. For some, Ultralente works like an intermediate-acting insulin, while for others it has a very long action.

A new once-a-day insulin released in May 2001 is Lantus (insulin glargine). Tests have shown that it is a true "peakless" insulin, providing 24-hour glucose-lowering activity with just one injection.

A fourth type of insulin became available in 1996, called Humalog, or insulin lispro. Humalog is a rapid-acting insulin, which begins to work five to ten minutes after it is injected, peaks in about one to two hours, and is gone in about three to five hours. This newer insulin acts much faster than regular insulin and can be injected just prior to a meal, rather than 30 minutes before a meal, which is recommended for regular insulin. Because it works so fast, it does a better job keeping blood glucose levels down right after eating. Also, because it is cleared from the body so quickly, there is less risk of hypoglycemia. Furthermore, because of Humalog's fast action, there is more flexibility in meal planning and timing—a true lifestyle benefit for people who must use insulin.

> ### Fast Fix
>
> Insulin lispro is a newer fast-acting insulin that can be injected just prior to a meal and so allows more flexibility in meal planning and timing.

The final type of insulin is *premixed insulin*. Premixed insulins consist of different insulins that are combined into fixed percentages. These insulins are convenient for some people who combine two different insulins together, such as NPH and regular. The most typical mixture is 70 percent NPH and 30 percent regular, called 70/30 insulin. Other mixtures that are available are 50/50 insulin, which is 50 percent NPH and 50 percent regular, and 75/25, a combination of 75 percent NPL (a long-acting form of Humalog insulin, only available in this mixture) and 25 percent Humalog.

Because premixed insulin preparations represent a combination of two different insulins, the onset, peak, and duration of these mixed insulins are a combination of the onset, peak, and duration of each individual insulin. This requires considerably more rigidity in your life, allowing for little variance in meal timing or amount of food eaten. Premixed insulin is best used by those unwilling or unable to take multiple injections each day, those unable or unwilling to test blood glucose levels frequently, those who have trouble drawing up insulin out of two different bottles, and those without the ability to adjust insulin dosing based on blood glucose readings. You are generally unable to achieve normal glucose control using premixed insulin, and the major goals of this type of insulin therapy are to prevent both low and very high blood glucose levels.

A Measure of Strength

Pure insulin is a very small, white crystal. When it is made into a solution, it is dissolved or suspended in a liquid. These liquid solutions have different strengths, and the strengths are measured in units of active insulin. The most common insulin available in the United States is U-100 insulin. A U-100 insulin has 100 units of active insulin in each milliliter (mL) of liquid. You can think of it as 100 pieces of insulin in each milliliter of liquid. Using your math skills, this would mean that there are 1,000 units of insulin (10 mL x 100 units/mL) in one 10-mL vial of insulin. Other concentrations of insulin, such as U-40, U-50, and U-500, are available, but they are rarely used in the United States today. In Europe and Latin America, U-40 can still be found in use, an important bit of information to know if you are a frequent international traveler.

Give It a Shot

Since insulin is a protein, it cannot be taken orally because the body's digestive juices would destroy it; it must be given by injection. The timing and frequency of insulin injections depend upon a number of factors, including the type of insulin, amount and type of food eaten, and the person's level of physical activity. By testing your blood glucose levels frequently and working together with your health care team to analyze your glucose patterns, you and your team will identify the right insulin "fit" for you.

Once your patterns are identified, you then need to choose the insulin delivery system that is right for you. Not too long ago, your only option was a glass syringe with its "sharpen after each use" detachable needle. As metal technology advanced, it was replaced by the disposable needle-and-syringe combination, which had a very sharp, very strong, yet significantly thinner (and thus less painful) needle. Today, syringe needles are so small that in most instances the injection is almost painless. You often need to look to make sure the needle is through the skin when giving yourself a shot. And when asked, most people who use insulin say that it is a much bigger deal, and more painful, to test your glucose than to administer an injection.

While syringes have greatly improved over the last 75 years, they still require the insulin to be drawn from a vial. This can be inconvenient for anyone attempting to lead a normal, active life, and studies have shown that miscalculated insulin doses are not uncommon. These concerns led to the development of insulin pens, which were first used in Europe and then introduced to the United States in the early 1990s. An insulin pen looks very similar to a fountain pen, except that insulin goes where you would normally find an ink cartridge and a needle replaces the point of the pen. Your insulin dose is then "dialed up" and the top is pressed down to deliver your insulin. Simplifying

(Continued on page 214)

Giving Yourself a Shot:
Preparing and Injecting the Insulin

WHAT YOU NEED TO DO	WHY YOU NEED TO DO IT
Look at the vial or cartridge of insulin before you use it.	Clumps that do not dissolve, color change, or cloudiness (of a clear insulin) means the insulin may be damaged and thus no good.
Check the expiration date of the insulin.	Old insulin has lost some of its effectiveness, and it will not work well or as expected.
If using a cloudy insulin, such as NPH or 70/30, gently roll the vial between the palms of your hands. If you are using an insulin pen, invert the pen 15 times to mix the insulin.	Cloudy insulin is a mixture of insulins and/or additives to prolong or change its action. If not mixed, you will receive an incorrect percentage of the insulin, in addition to changing the percentage of remaining insulin.
Wash hands and clean your injection site.	This prevents infection.

Use a new syringe or new pen needle each time.	This prevents infection. In addition, new needles are sharp. Dull needles hurt.
If using a vial, first draw up air equal to your dose, then inject this air into the vial.	This fills the vial with pressure to help with the withdrawal of insulin.
Turn the vial upside down, and withdraw more than the number of units you need, then push up to the amount you need.	This prevents bubbles in the syringe.
If using an insulin pen, once you attach a new needle to the pen, prime the pen with a two-unit shot into the air, then dial up your dose.	This assures that the pen is delivering insulin and fills the needle with insulin in preparation for injecting the proper dose.
Pinch the skin, push the needle straight in, and push the plunger down. Count to five before removing the needle.	This allows for complete delivery of the insulin and prevents insulin from leaking out of the injection site.
Stop pinching and remove the needle.	CONGRATULATIONS & WELL DONE!

the process has increased compliance with frequent injections (especially those during the middle of the day, when the person is likely to be away from home) and increased the accuracy of delivered doses. Insulin pens come in two sizes, with 150- or 300-unit cartridges, and in most types of insulin: regular, Humalog, NPH, premixed 70/30 and 50/50, and Humalog Mixed 75/25.

Pen Ease

The development of the insulin pen helped increase compliance and remedy the common problem of mis-measured insulin doses.

Despite these advances and the improved compliance they've brought, there are still several bumps in the road to tighter glucose control. The first "bump" is the difficulty in accurately matching the peak-time variability of the intermediate- and long-acting insulins with the rise in glucose levels you have first thing in the morning. This is called the *dawn phenomenon* and is caused by your liver increasing its glucose output every night at about 3 A.M. in preparation for the coming day. In order to accurately match your insulin needs, it would be best not to take any long-acting insulin at all but rather to get up at 3 A.M. every night to inject regular insulin to correct for this condition.

Since that doesn't make for a very good long-term treatment plan, the longer lasting insulins are the best alternative.

The second problem occurs when the rate of insulin absorption does not match the glucose rise after meals. This variation can result from the sites you select for injection or the repeated use of a favorite site. Absorption of insulin is dependent upon where you inject it. Insulin injections in the stomach act faster than injections in your arm, injections in your arm act faster than those in your leg, and injections in the buttocks are slowest acting of all. The blood flow to the injection site also governs absorption, so that cold skin makes for slower absorption than does warm skin. Blood flow is also changed when injections are continually given at the same site, because excessive insulin in one area promotes the growth of fat tissue, called *lipohypertrophy*. This fat tissue has few blood vessels and, therefore, absorbs insulin poorly. By changing injection sites (pick a spot about one inch from the last injection site), you can generally prevent this problem.

Finally, your daytime, base insulin need is sometimes difficult to match. Your base insulin need, also called your basal, is what your body requires to function when you are in a fasting state between meals. The same variation that is associated with the dawn phenomenon occurs in some people in a milder form during the day as well.

To address these problems and to meet the needs of people desiring the best glucose control possible, the late 1970s saw the introduction of the insulin pump, which provided continuous delivery of regular insulin directly under the skin. Unfortunately, the first pumps were not very reliable. By the 1990s, the kinks had been ironed out and the pumps improved so dramatically that they are currently considered the best method for delivering insulin in almost all people who require insulin. The number of people on pumps in the United States has risen from 20,000 in 1995 to over 80,000 in 1999. This number is climbing and increasing by over 20,000 new pumpers each year.

These modern pumps are quite similar to the IV machines used in hospitals to deliver medication, only much smaller. They are usually the size of a beeper and weigh about four ounces. Each pump has a thin plastic tube, with one end connected to the insulin reservoir inside the pump and the other end to a thin plastic catheter. This catheter is generally placed under the skin of your abdomen using an insertion needle, which is removed once the catheter is in place. The catheter site is changed every two to three days. That means that instead of requiring 8 to 12 insulin injections over the course of two to three days, you need only one needle injection, to place the catheter, during the same time period if you use a pump. Your insulin pump is then programmed to deliver insulin at a specific rate throughout the day and night (your basal rate) to compensate for the dawn phenomenon and your daytime base needs. This

Pump Up

Modern insulin pumps are considered the best way to deliver insulin in almost all who require it.

leaves you free to eat at any time, and you are no longer tied to the timing of insulin injections, which significantly reduces the risk of hypoglycemia. Each time you eat, you simply direct the pump to deliver a bolus (or added amount) of insulin to match the amount of food you want to eat.

But there are downsides to the pump. One of the major drawbacks is the risk of infection at the insertion site. This is usually remedied by making sure that the site is changed often enough and that a good, clean insertion technique is used. Other quite serious problems are the very high glucose levels and even life-threatening ketoacidosis that can occur if insulin delivery is disrupted for longer than a few hours. This can happen if the pump malfunctions, the tubing becomes kinked or blocked, or the pump runs out of insulin. With all the bells and whistles available on today's pumps, however, a vigilant user is likely to notice such a pump problem before insulin delivery is disrupted for any serious length of time.

The last two hurdles tend to be cost (a pump costs about $6,000) and the issue of constantly being "hooked up" to something. While the cost of a pump is daunting, the cost of keeping an individual with diabetes well is far less than treating someone with complications. Many insurance companies are becoming more aware of this and are beginning to find that the cost of the pump far outweighs the long-term costs of someone in poor health and poor control. For this reason, with prior authorization, many insurance companies, including MediCare, do cover insulin pumps.

Finally, the issue of attachment is usually fast to fade. Pumps are so small that they are easily slipped into your pocket, clipped onto your belt, or hidden under your clothes. Just check out pictures of Nicole Johnson, Miss America 1998, in her evening gown. Insulin dependent, she had her pump on during all but the swimsuit competition.

New Directions, New Delivery Systems

To avoid insulin injections, various delivery methods have been tried and used but with limited, if any, success. Mechanical devices, called jet injectors, use compressed air to blow the insulin under the skin. They have proved to be expensive, are bulky, and can still be painful, even more so than syringes. Nasal insulin was tried, but without success due to irritation of the mucous membranes of the nose. And the use of rectal insulin suppositories before meals has proved not to be socially acceptable for widespread use.

Holding the most promise is an inhaled aerosol spray that is proving to be as effective as injections. These inhaled-insulin delivery systems are currently being tested by at least three manufacturers. With these systems, packages of insulin become airborne in an enclosed cavity and are then inhaled. Much to the surprise of many diabetes experts, the inhaled insulin is rapidly absorbed and is not toxic to the lungs. One drawback is that the insulin lasts for less than an hour, so it could only be used for meal-insulin administration. The current systems are also bulky and require a lot of insulin to achieve the same effect as an injection. Still, large studies are underway with hopes of FDA approval in the near future.

Other promising avenues of investigation are the use of ultrasound pulses to deliver insulin through skin patches; implanted, extended-release insulin pellets; and an oral form of insulin. While oral insulin is really a misnomer, researchers have discovered a plantlike substance that can be taken orally and that appears to have effects similar to insulin. Trials are underway but findings from these studies are not expected until 2002 or later.

New disposable insulin pumps should be on the market in 2001. These look like patches and are applied to the body every three days. They will deliver insulin at a constant rate, so they would not be useful for correcting the dawn phenomenon or basal rate changes. Implantable pumps have been available for years but seem to be advancing in use very slowly. A very high insulin concentration (U-400) is delivered at set bolus (for after meals) and basal (ongoing) rates and is programmed using an external remote control. The pump needs to be refilled about every three months and, up until recently, was plagued by incidents of blockage in the delivery catheter. Reformulations of the insulin being delivered through these pumps seem to have improved the blockage situation. By combining this implantable pump with an implantable glucose sensor, the diabetes loop would be closed, creating a "mechanical" cure for diabetes. Such a system may become reality as soon as 2005.

Meanwhile, an exciting breakthrough in islet cell transplant research was developed in Canada and is being tested at medical centers in the United States. Researchers have demonstrated a possible cure for Type 1 diabetes, with people remaining insulin independent, with normal glucose levels, for up to two years, without significant side effects or complications. This, coupled with discoveries by California researchers who have been able to grow beta cells, resulting in an unlimited source of transplant material, may foretell an end to insulin-dependent diabetes.

Even though insulin is not a cure for diabetes, the 1922 medical discovery saved, and continues to save, millions of lives around the world. And while this Nobel-prize-winning accomplishment is among one of the greatest medical achievements, outside the Sir Frederick G. Banting Square at the Banting Museum in London, Ontario, still burns the Flame of Hope. Only when a cure, rather than a treatment, for diabetes is found will the flame be extinguished.

CHAPTER 12

Combination Therapy

T**he new drugs to treat diabetes have certainly changed the face of treatment. Each, alone, helps to fix a trouble spot in the diabetes process. But these individual tools in the expanding diabetes tool kit are increasingly being used in various combinations to make diabetes treatment more individualized—and more successful.**

Meeting More of Your Diabetes Needs

You're driving down that old diabetes road again. To keep moving, you must continue to put gas in your car. A bit down the road, you develop a very slow leak in one of your tires. Gas won't fix this problem. Every few hours, you must stop and fill the tire with air in order to keep moving, and you must continue to fill the car with gas as well. All of a sudden, your engine temperature light flashes. You pull the car over and discover a small hole in your radiator, and neither air nor gas will

Where Do They Work?

	GLITAZONES:	BIGUANIDE:	AGIS:	MEGLITINIDE:	SULFONYL-UREAS:
Type of Medication	Actos Avandia	Glucophage	Precose Glyset	Prandin	Micronase Diabeta Glynase Glucotrol Amaryl
Site of Action and Metabolic Effect	**FAT CELLS** Cause fat cells to take up more fatty acids and glucose, decreasing insulin resistance in the muscles	**LIVER** Causes liver to produce less glucose	**SMALL INTESTINE** Delay absorption of glucose in small intestine	**PANCREAS** Stimulates the beta cells to make more insulin	**PANCREAS** Stimulate the beta cells to make more insulin

fix this problem. You put in some water and get on your way, stopping every so often to add water to the radiator, air to the tires, and gas to the tank. While stopping and taking care of business is a hassle, as long as you continue this process your car drives beautifully and you get to where you are going safely.

Combining different diabetes medications together is very similar to fixing multiple automobile problems. In diabetes, you have multiple problems that need to be fixed, and not just one pill can meet every need. First, your muscles are not taking up the glucose in your bloodstream. Next, the liver is overproducing glucose, further increasing the glucose levels in your blood. And finally, the insulin production by your pancreas cannot keep up with the high levels of glucose in your blood. Different types of medication address these different concerns, and sometimes the combination of medications is even more effective in lowering glucose levels than a single pill is.

The One-Problem-at-a-Time Approach

In the United States, up until five years ago, there was little discussion of multiple-medication therapy for people with diabetes. The only "combination therapy" was the addition of insulin to a maximum dose of a sulfonylurea, if and when the pills alone could not get the job done. With the release of four new types of medications in the past few years, there are now more than 30 different combinations of medications that can used for the treatment of diabetes.

The most commonly used method of introducing medications to improve glucose control is called the "Step System." Medications are slowly and systematically added, with the goal of achieving glucose control. Because the glitazones address the primary problem in Type 2 diabetes—insulin resistance—and because there is no risk of hypo-glycemia with them, they are the best first-line treatment. The next step of glucose control adds Glucophage, for its additional effect on the liver and, again, its lack of hypoglycemia potential. If glucose levels continue to increase, the addition of a sulfonylurea or Prandin may be necessary. Acarbose is occasionally used either prior to or after the addition of a sulfonylurea, but its use in the United States is limited. The final addition is insulin. The Step System, sometimes also referred to as the "Stutter System," usually fails to work because it just never seems to catch up to the rising glucose levels. It is a slow approach, and sometimes the doses are not increased fast enough, keeping glucose levels elevated for months before a dose increase or additional med-ication is tried.

The Total Overhaul

The reality for most people when they first develop diabetes, or when they finally decide that they need to take care of themselves, is that their glucose levels are generally quite high. One med-ication will rarely make the grade. Glucose levels are in a toxic range, the pancreas can't keep up, and the cell resistance to insulin is astronomical.

(Continued on page 228)

Can They Work Together?

TYPE OF MEDICATION	BIGUANIDE	AGIs	MEGLITINIDE	SULFONYLUREAS	INSULIN
Glitazones Actos Avandia	Great combination. Lowers glucose output by liver and increases glucose uptake by the muscles. No hypoglycemia.	Slight benefit. Increases glucose uptake by the muscles and improves after-meal glucose levels. No hypoglycemia.	Probably good, but few studies. Increases glucose uptake by muscles; stimulates release of insulin at meals. Small risk of hypoglycemia.	Good combination. Increases glucose uptake by muscles; stimulates release of insulin throughout the day. Risk of hypoglycemia.	Good combination. Glitazone added to insulin reduces the amount of insulin. Risk of hypoglycemia.
Biguanide Glucophage		Slight benefit. Decreases glucose output by liver and improves after-meal glucose levels.	Probably good, few studies. Decreases glucose output by liver; stimulates release of insulin at meals. Small risk of hypoglycemia.	Good combination. Decreases glucose output by liver, stimulates release of insulin throughout day. Risk of hypoglycemia.	Good, but not as beneficial as insulin combined with glitazone. Risk of hypoglycemia.
Meglitinide Prandin				No reason to use both together.	Pills at meals and NPH insulin at bedtime. Stimulates release of insulin at meals and maintains basal insulin at night. Risk of hypoglycemia.

TYPE OF MEDICATION	BIGUANIDE	AGIs	MEGLITINIDE	SULFONYLUREAS	INSULIN
Alpha Gluco-sidase Inhibitors (AGIs) Precose Glyset			Probably good, but few studies done. Stimulates release of insulin at meals and improves after-meal glucose levels. Small risk of hypoglycemia; must be treated with glucose tabs.	Good combination. Stimulates release of insulin throughout day and improves after-meal glucose levels. Risk of hypoglycemia; must be treated with glucose tabs.	Possible combination, but no studies done. Improves after-meal glucose levels. Risk of hypoglycemia; must be treated with glucose tabs.
Sulfonylureas Micronase Diabeta Glynase Glucotrol Amaryl					Pills during day and NPH insulin at bedtime. Stimulates release of insulin at meals and maintains basal insulin needs at night. Risk of hypoglycemia.

The "Blast and Taper Fast System" temporarily forces the pancreas to make more insulin, decreases glucose output by the liver, and addresses the insulin resistance

caused by the continuously high glucose levels. In this approach, a glitazone such as Actos or Avandia is started to decrease insulin resistance, Glucophage is given to decrease the glucose output by the liver, and a sulfonylurea, such as Glucotrol, or the meglitinide Prandin is used to stimulate the beta cells and increase insulin production. Insulin may even be used early on in this approach. Blood glucose levels are checked frequently (four times per day), and as soon as the glucose levels begin to fall below 120 mg/dl, the insulin and sulfonylurea or meglitinide doses are decreased rapidly and may even be stopped as goal glucose levels are achieved. As the glitazone takes its full effect, if glucose levels become normal, Glucophage may even be decreased or discontinued as well, as long as the blood glucose remains below 120 mg/dl.

The goal with the Blast and Taper Fast System is to use the maximum dose and number of medications to achieve the maximum control as soon as possible. Once glucose levels begin to respond and before hypoglycemia becomes an issue, medications are quickly tapered off, starting with any that can cause hypoglycemia, allowing the long-term beneficial effects of the glitazones to continue. In this way, even those whose diabetes is sorely out of control can begin to improve their condition and lower the risk of complications.

Either Way, Get It Fixed!

Always remember that high glucose levels are extremely toxic. Your body cannot tolerate them—nor should you. Don't count your pills and feel that you've failed. It is not the number of pills you take, but rather the glucose levels you achieve, the complications you prevent, and the joyful life you lead that determines your diabetes success.

Organizations

American Association of Diabetes Educators
100 West Monroe Street, Suite 400
Chicago, IL 60603-1901
800-832-6874
http://www.aadenet.org

The American Association of Diabetes Educators is
an organization of health professionals who teach
people with diabetes. You can contact the Association for a referral to a diabetes educator near you.

American Diabetes Association
National Office
1701 North Beauregard Street
Alexandria, VA 22311
800-342-2383
http://www.diabetes.org

The aim of the American Diabetes Association is "to
prevent and cure diabetes and to improve the lives of
all people affected by diabetes." By calling the phone
number listed above, you can access the Association's Diabetes Information and Action Line, which
is staffed by trained operators who can provide
information on diabetes management and refer you
to local diabetes programs and services, including
education classes, support groups, and advocacy
services. The Association's Web site also provides
an abundance of information on diabetes risk, nutrition, exercise, news, management tips, and more.

Additional Diabetes Web Resources

Diabetes 1 2 3
http://www.diabetes123.com

This attractive site provides basic information for
kids, parents, and adults with diabetes. It also allows

you to ask questions of an experienced team of diabetes professionals.

Diabetes.com
http://www.diabetes.com

This consumer-friendly site offers a diabetes library, the latest diabetes health news, message boards, and a weekly chat. The Health Library is loaded with easy-to-read, enlightening articles on diet, exercise, intimacy, avoiding complications, and other practical concerns of people with diabetes.

DiabetesWebSite.com
http://www.diabeteswebsite.com

This site, with its neighborly feel, offers solid information on diabetes and helpful advice on living well with the disease, including tips on travel, exercise, emotions, intimacy, and even diabetes etiquette.

DiabeticCooking.com
http://www.DiabeticCooking.com

This easy-to-use Web site allows you to search hundreds of recipes specially selected for people with diabetes. The recipes come complete with nutrition information.

Joslin Diabetes Center
http://www.joslin.harvard.edu

The Joslin Diabetes Center, associated with Harvard Medical School, is a leader in diabetes research, treatment, and education. Its site provides news, a library, online discussions, and information on participating in clinical research programs.

Rick Mendosa's Diabetes Directory
http://www.mendosa.com/diabetes.htm

Rick Mendosa has been tracking online diabetes resources since 1995. His directory of "On-line Diabetes Resources" provides descriptions and addresses of a vast array of diabetes-related pages on the Web, including those from organizations, universities, hospitals, research institutions, and the government. Also included are listings for diabetes publications on the Web; company sites; sites in languages other than English; and sites devoted to diabetes medications, software, glucose meters, and diabetic neuropathy.

National Institute of Diabetes and Digestive and Kidney Diseases (NIDDK)
http://www.niddk.nih.gov

The NIDDK is part of the U.S. Government's National Institutes of Health. Its Web site is packed with health information for people with diabetes. Click on "Diabetes" under the Health Information heading for a long list of online publications, resources, and links covering everything from diagnosing diabetes to alternative therapies and targeted material for high-risk groups such as African- and Hispanic-Americans. You'll find links to other resources, including the National Diabetes Information Clearinghouse, the National Diabetes Education Program, and a directory of diabetes organizations. And you can find out about clinical research and participation in clinical trials.

Additional Health Resources

American Cancer Society
800-227-2345
http://www.cancer.org

Contact the American Cancer Society to learn more about the dangers of smoking and for information and advice on how to quit.

American Dietetic Association
216 West Jackson Boulevard, Suite 800
Chicago, IL 60606

Consumer Nutrition Hotline: 800-366-1655
http://www.eatright.org

In addition to providing a medley of information on nutrition, the American Dietetic Association can refer you to a dietitian in your area who specializes in the counseling of people with diabetes.

American Heart Association
National Center
7272 Greenville Avenue
Dallas, TX 75231
800-242-8721
http://www.americanheart.org

For information on preventing, detecting, and treating heart disease, high blood pressure, and stroke, all of which are more common in people with diabetes, contact the American Heart Association. You can also visit the Association's inviting, user-friendly Web site for a variety of tips and recommendations.

American Lung Association
800-586-4872
http://www.lungusa.org

The American Lung Association can provide you with information and advice that will help you quit smoking.

National Kidney Foundation
30 East 33rd Street, Suite 1100
New York, NY 10016
800-622-9010
http://www.kidney.org

The Foundation can provide you with information on kidney disease and kidney transplants.